RAND NATIONAL DEFENSE RESEARCH INSTITUTE

T0303160

The Air Force Deployment Transition Center

Assessment of Program Structure, Process, and Outcomes

Terry L. Schell, Coreen Farris, Jeremy N. V. Miles, Jennifer Sloan,
Deborah M. Scharf

Prepared for Office of the Secretary of Defense and the Defense Centers of Excellence for Psychological Health and Traumatic Brain Injury

For more information on this publication, visit www.rand.org/t/RR918

Library of Congress Cataloging-in-Publication Data
ISBN: 978-0-8330-9540-4

Published by the RAND Corporation, Santa Monica, Calif.

Preface

It is often accepted as common knowledge that military personnel benefit from decompression time between a war zone and the home station. With the ubiquity of air travel, it is now possible for service members to leave an active conflict zone and be greeted by their families within a matter of hours. Some within the military mental health community have argued that service members would have better post-deployment behavioral health outcomes if they had more time to process their experiences between leaving the war zone and returning to friends, families, and civilian settings. To capitalize on the potential benefits of a decompression period paired with support services, the U.S. Air Force established the Deployment Transition Center (DTC) at Ramstein Air Base in Germany in July 2010.

The DTC provides airmen returning from combat missions with an opportunity to decompress and share lessons learned before returning to their home stations. The program length is four days, during which service members have an opportunity to debrief their experiences with fellow airmen and receive structured reintegration support during group sessions. During this time, DTC participants are encouraged to get adequate rest, and DTC staff handle such details as transportation arrangements to remove as many inconveniences and stressors as possible.

To identify benefits associated with the DTC and lessons for similar programs across the U.S. Department of Defense, the Defense Centers of Excellence for Psychological Health and Traumatic Brain Injury (DCoE) asked RAND researchers to evaluate the structure, processes, and outcomes of the program.

This research was sponsored by DCoE and conducted within the Forces and Resources Policy Center of the RAND National Defense Research Institute, a federally funded research and development center sponsored by the Office of the Secretary of Defense, the Joint Staff, the Unified Combatant Commands, the Navy, the Marine Corps, the defense agencies, and the defense Intelligence Community. For more information on the RAND Forces and Resources Policy Center, see www.rand.org/nsrd/ndri/centers/frp or contact the director (contact information is provided on the web page).

This report is one of a series of program evaluations conducted as part of the "Innovative Practices for Psychological Health and Traumatic Brain Injury" project; for more information and to access other products from this project, please visit the project web page: www.rand.org/multi/military/innovative-practices.

Contents

Figures and Tables

Figures

Tables

Summary

Following the Falklands War in 1982, United Kingdom military personnel returned from their deployments in one of two ways: entirely by sea or by a combination of sea and air travel. Those who returned entirely by sea had journeys that were one week longer than those who split their mode of travel. Press reports at the time suggested that those who spent longer getting home had better psychological outcomes than those who made the trip more quickly. Although outcome data to substantiate that claim have never surfaced, the narrative has entered into legend and is widely cited in support for providing decompression time between a war zone and home station.

Today, with the ubiquity of air travel, it is possible for service members to leave an active conflict zone and be greeted by their families within a matter of hours. Would these service members have better outcomes if they had more decompression time before returning to friends, families, and civilian settings? To capitalize on the potential benefits of a decompression period paired with support services, the U.S. Air Force established the Deployment Transition Center (DTC) at Ramstein Air Base in Germany in July 2010. The DTC provides airmen returning home from combat missions with an opportunity to decompress and share lessons learned before returning to their home stations. The program length is four days, during which service members receive an opportunity to debrief with fellow airmen and structured reintegration support during group sessions. During this time, DTC participants are encouraged to get adequate rest, and DTC staff handle such details as transportation arrangements to remove as many inconveniences and stressors as possible.

Ramstein Air Base serves as a "third location" (i.e., neither conflict zone nor home base), a neutral setting in which returning trauma-exposed airmen can focus on reintegration without the stressors of a conflict zone or the stimuli of civilian life, including the demands of family and friends. Ramstein was identified as a safe, peaceful setting in which to adjust slowly to and prepare for reintegration. The agricultural fields and mixed forests of southwestern Germany may feel more familiar to many Americans than the climate and geography of Iraq or Afghanistan, and the foreign location maintains a significant geographic separation from most family members and friends.

The DTC identified "decompression" as a theoretical construct that promotes a healthy psychological response to deployment trauma. According to program materials, decompression has three elements: (1) *rest and relaxation (R&R)*, (2) *debriefing* adverse events experienced during the deployment, and (3) *preparing for reintegration* with family and friends by reviewing adaptive and maladaptive psychosocial coping strategies. Most elements of the DTC, from logistical support to its formal curriculum, are intended to contribute to one or more of these decompression elements. The DTC also focuses on collecting and sharing lessons learned during attendees' just-completed deployments. This is intended to help the Air Force identify policies and procedures that could improve mission effectiveness in theater. Airmen participate in group sessions led by a recently deployed Air Force facilitator in the same career field as the group. The information collected by the facilitator may be used to fine-tune the deployment process, training, or support of service members in the career field. Figure S.1 shows the typical program schedule.

Attendance at the DTC is limited to airmen who were regularly exposed to significant risk of death in direct combat or regularly exposed to traumatic events during their deployment. At the time of this report, all members of four mission sets with high degrees of exposure to the risk of injury or death are preselected to attend: security forces, explosive ordinance disposal, tactical air control parties, and convoy operators. Other individuals or teams of airmen can be nominated by a deployed commander to attend the DTC if they experienced unanticipated or repeated exposure to trauma. DTC staff members estimate that approximately half of program participants are members of pre-identified mission sets, and half are command-nominated.

The goal of the DTC is to provide airmen with the skills necessary for successful psychosocial adjustment following their return to their home stations, workplaces, and families (e.g., adaptive coping mechanisms, knowledge of military mental health resources). However, in outward-facing materials, the program purposely avoids pointing to behavioral health outcomes as its primary goal. This ensures that DTC participants do not perceive the program as mental health treatment, which reduces stigma-related barriers to actively participating and benefiting from the program. Nonetheless, the outcomes selected for an internal Air Force evaluation, briefings on the program, and our communication with program leaders suggest that a reduction in post-deployment posttraumatic stress disorder (PTSD), depression symptoms, and alcohol misuse are important program targets. Relatedly, the DTC recruits a group of airmen who are at high risk for psychiatric disorders and includes in its curriculum structured program elements that were originally designed for the purpose of reducing psychiatric symptoms or psychological distress (Adler et al., 2009).

Figure S.1
Schedule and Goals of DTC Groups and Activities

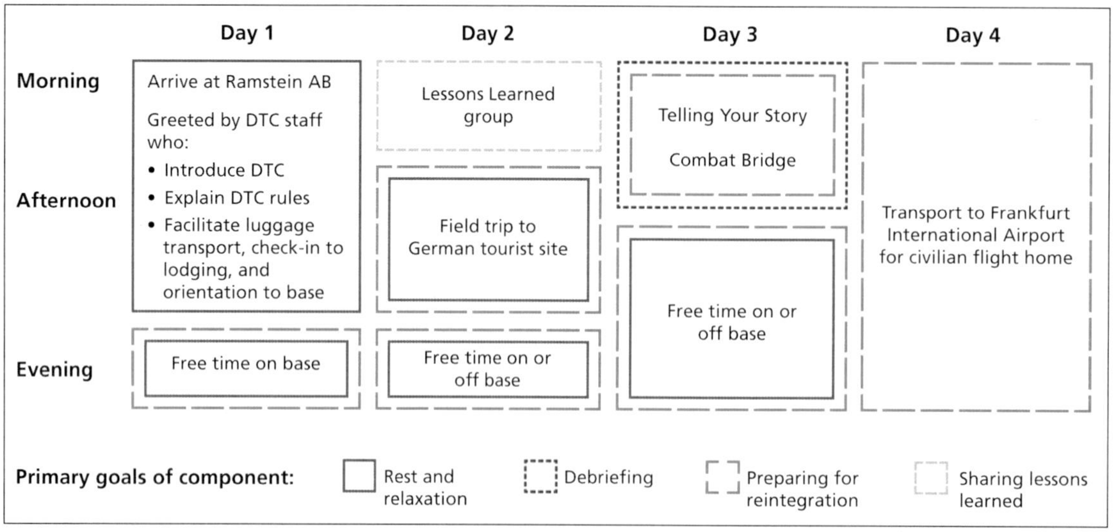

RAND *RR918-S.1*

Evaluation Approach

The Defense Centers for Excellence in Psychological Health and Traumatic Brain Injury contracted with RAND to complete an evaluation of the DTC that would

- document and evaluate the structure and processes of the DTC program
- assess attendee satisfaction with the program
- evaluate post-deployment outcomes.

Our approach to achieving these aims included (1) a site visit that included interviews with DTC leadership and staff, (2) a review of DTC program materials, (3) a literature review of interventions for individuals with trauma exposure, (4) review and summary of DTC-collected participant satisfaction data, and (5) an analysis of post-deployment outcomes as measured by the U.S. Department of Defense (DoD)-administered Post-Deployment Health Re-Assessment (PDHRA).

To document the structure and processes associated with the DTC, we visited the program site at Ramstein Air Base in Germany. While there, we toured the facilities and interviewed program leadership and staff members. To protect the privacy of airmen attending the program, we did not meet with attendees or observe groups. We used the information we gathered during the site visit and interviews, supplemented with information from the program concept of operations (U.S. Air Forces in Europe, 2014), to document the structure and processes of the program.

To review benefits associated with the DTC and lessons for similar programs across DoD, we reviewed the literature on programs and interventions for individuals who have experienced a traumatic event that sought to prevent the development of lasting mental health problems. We used this review to identify programs that are similar to the DTC and to summarize their evidence base. We first reviewed the small but growing literature on third-location decompression (TLD) programs, which most closely match the DTC's program structure. Second, we reviewed the small body of research on non-TLD programs aimed at armed forces personnel. The selected programs included either debriefing or psychoeducational strategies to reduce the likelihood of mental health problems post-deployment. These programs did not include an R&R component. Finally, we turned to the methodologically rigorous body of work on PTSD prevention among civilians exposed to traumatic events. Although lessons from such programs may not be perfectly aligned with programs serving military populations, their outcomes provided a starting point for evaluation and helped to guide expectations regarding the DTC's outcomes.

We supplemented our literature review with a review of program participants' responses to an anonymous satisfaction survey administered to airmen at the end of their DTC stay. This survey was designed and administered by DTC program staff. The survey contained four sections. The first queried attendees' opinions of the DTC overall, specific program content, and perceived skills and readiness to reintegrate with family and friends. The second section assessed respondents' current well-being, including perceived physical fitness, psychological well-being, and work-related quality of life. The third section included two questions about religious services, and the final section of the survey used open-ended questions to assess what each participant (1) liked about the DTC, (2) disliked about the DTC, and (3) would change about the DTC.

Finally, we assessed the difference between DTC attendees and a comparison group of similar airmen who did not attend the DTC. All outcomes were assessed using data available on the DoD-administered PDHRA questionnaire, given three to six months after return from deployment. We identified four measures on this assessment that map to some of the primary DTC program goals: PTSD symptoms, depressive symptoms, binge drinking, and social conflicts with family and coworkers. Using individual participant identifiers and attendance dates for DTC attendees, we compared DTC attendees with a matched control group on the four available and relevant outcomes. Matching was done on the basis of airman and deployment characteristics that were assessed on the Post-Deployment Health Assessment (PDHA), a mandatory survey given within 30 days of the end of the deployment.

Key Findings

Lessons from Similar Programs

Our review of TLD program evaluations identified no high-quality randomized controlled trials, but there are published studies on program implementation and participant satisfaction. These studies revealed high levels of participant satisfaction with TLD programs. We also identified a prior study of the DTC itself, which indicated that fewer DTC participants reported at least one PTSD symptom following a deployment (14.1 percent) compared with nonparticipants (23.4 percent; Wirick, Garb, and Dickey, 2012). According to this study, airmen who attended the DTC were also less likely to screen positive for alcohol misuse at follow-up than airmen who did not attend.

Components of TLD programs can be implemented without requiring a third location. That is, service members may participate in debriefing sessions or receive psychoeducation about mental health symptoms and family reintegration on return to their home station instead of at a third location. The documented outcomes of these practices are mixed (Mulligan, Fear, et al., 2011a), with some programs demonstrating positive outcomes for those with high combat exposure (Adler et al., 2009), and others failing to show a positive impact associated with the program (e.g., Deahl et al., 1994).

We highlight one particular evaluation of a reintegration program for its direct relevance to the DTC. Adler and colleagues (2009) conducted a randomized controlled trial of Battlemind, a debriefing program—delivered at a home station—that provides an opportunity to reflect on deployment experiences and discuss the transition from combat to home. The DTC uses revised training materials from this program for its Combat Bridge session. The evaluation showed that soldiers who attended Battlemind had fewer PTSD, depression, and sleep symptoms four months after the intervention than those who did not attend, but these reductions were true only among those who had high levels of combat exposure (Adler et al., 2009). Moreover, the size of this effect, even among those with high combat exposure, was small. For example, soldiers who received the Battlemind debriefing scored three points lower on the PTSD Checklist (Weathers et al., 1993), a drop that is not considered to be a clinically significant change (Monson et al., 2008; National Center for PTSD, 2012).

In addition to evaluations of military-specific reintegration programs, it also possible to glean insight from civilian programs designed to prevent the development of mental health problems following exposure to a trauma. We reviewed the outcomes of PTSD prevention programs that share commonalities with the DTC.

Psychological debriefing is a group-based intervention in which survivors of a shared trauma describe and relive the trauma in detail with the expectation that emotional catharsis or ventilation will prevent development of more severe trauma symptomatology. A systematic review of the extensive literature on posttraumatic debriefing concluded that individuals exposed to psychological debriefing programs are just as likely to develop PTSD as individuals who do not participate (Rose et al., 2002). In fact, two rigorous evaluations found that debriefing was associated with an *increased* risk of PTSD (Bisson et al., 1997; Hobbs et al., 1996). At this date, researchers and clinical practice guidelines recommend that civilian-style debriefing programs not be offered to trauma survivors (U.S. Department of Veterans Affairs and U.S. Department of Defense, 2010; McNally, Bryant, and Ehlers, 2003; Nash and Watson, 2011; Rose et al., 2002). Because the DTC includes program elements that are similar to those used in critical incident stress debriefing, it is likely that those particular elements are contraindicated by existing DoD and U.S. Department of Veterans Affairs treatment guidelines.

An alternative to providing prevention services to all trauma-exposed individuals is to provide services only to those who have begun to develop traumatic stress symptoms (but who have not yet developed PTSD). The best-studied and most widely disseminated intervention for early trauma symptoms is trauma-focused cognitive behavioral therapy (TF-CBT), a brief, four- to five-session therapy that includes education about stress responses to trauma, habituation to the trauma memory, real-world exposures to safe but avoided situations, and cognitive therapy to modify maladaptive beliefs associated with the trauma (U.S. Department of Veterans Affairs and U.S. Department of Defense, 2010; McNally, Bryant, and Ehlers, 2003). Trauma-exposed individuals who have posttraumatic psychological symptoms and who receive TF-CBT are less likely to develop PTSD (Roberts et al., 2009).

Lessons from Participant Experiences

Airmen who attended the DTC were invited on the last day of the program to complete a satisfaction survey. The survey was designed and administered by DTC staff. The DTC shared with the RAND research team aggregate survey results from 1,552 DTC attendees. Given that the data were shared in de-identified and aggregate form, we are unable to describe associations between attendee characteristics (gender, rank, or deployment experience) and satisfaction with the program. Nonetheless, the survey data provide a general picture of airmen's experiences at the DTC and their general subjective states as they prepared to return home.

Eighty percent of attendees reported that the DTC was a worthwhile experience, and three-quarters indicated that it helped prepare them to return home. In open-field portions of the survey, attendees reported that they liked the DTC accommodations, particularly the rooms in which they stayed, noting that the generous accommodations contributed to the perceived effectiveness of the DTC. Among those offering comments on the DTC's location, views were mixed. About half commented positively (49 percent) about being in Germany, but 31 percent had negative opinions about the distance between their living quarters and other buildings on the base, such as restaurants or the gym.

In general, respondents rated the DTC's classroom modules highly, with approximately two-thirds or more agreeing that each program module was helpful and increased reintegration knowledge and skills. Similarly, the majority indicated that the length of the program was "just right."

The survey also asked DTC attendees to describe their current well-being, including perceived physical health, emotional well-being, and work-related quality of life. In general, respondents indicated that their well-being and work-related quality of life were good and that the DTC had facilitated their ability to relax. More than 90 percent of participating airmen believed they had the skills to return home, and 87 percent said that they were emotionally prepared to reintegrate.

Negative comments were generally in the areas of transportation, program rules (such as alcohol limits and curfews), and mandatory attendance at the DTC. There were numerous suggestions to improve the shuttle system. There were also suggestions to revisit the protocol for selecting DTC attendees, including making attendance optional or taking into consideration whether an airman saw combat during the deployment. Other suggestions included making the field trip outside Ramstein optional and improving communication leading up to DTC stays, such as what to expect and what to bring.

Lessons from Quantitative Assessment of Program Outcomes

To evaluate the outcomes associated with DTC attendance, we conducted a propensity score analysis to estimate the effect of program attendance on PTSD symptoms, depressive symptoms, alcohol use, and family/work conflict following a deployment. The gold standard in evaluating an intervention is the randomized controlled trial, in which individuals who are eligible for a program are randomly assigned to either the intervention or control group. However, all eligible airmen who were able to attend the program did so, precluding a traditional randomized controlled trial. The propensity score analysis attempts to achieve the type of balance between comparison groups that is achieved with random assignment even when random assignment is not possible. We used propensity score–based analyses to compare DTC attendees with a group of similar airmen who did not attend the DTC. All background variables used for propensity matching were taken from the mandatory PDHA administered within 30 days of redeployment (i.e., return from deployment), including demographic factors, career field, deployment characteristics (e.g., length, combat exposure), physical injuries, and deployment trauma. We compared DTC attendees with the matched control group on four outcomes measured in the PDHRA administered 90–180 days after DTC attendance: PTSD symptoms, depressive symptoms, alcohol use, and conflicts with family and coworkers.

We controlled for demographic differences between groups using propensity weights to the extent possible, but some differences remained significant and may have posed a threat to the validity of the study. To avoid biases caused by these imbalances, we estimated treatment effects while including statistical covariates (i.e., doubly robust estimates). Specifically, we included as covariates variables that were significantly different across groups even after propensity weighting. We also included covariates when that variable was a strong predictor of our outcomes of interest.

The differences in key outcomes between DTC participants and their historical controls (i.e., matched airmen who completed their deployments before the DTC was available and, therefore, did not attend) were small and not statistically significant for PTSD symptom counts, frequency of depressive symptoms, and incidence of social conflict. For binge drinking, the mean for the DTC attendees was approximately 25 percent lower than that for the control group. To assess historical trends, we examined these outcomes over time among airmen who were not sent to the DTC and were not in the control group. There were no significant trends in PTSD, depression, or social conflict observed in the airmen who did not attend the DTC over this period. However, there was a significant reduction in post-deployment binge drinking observed over this time period even for those airmen who did not attend the DTC.

This historical trend toward less alcohol use across the entire Air Force fully accounted for the observed difference in alcohol use when comparing DTC attendees to their historical controls (i.e., the DTC added no beneficial effect over and above the changes seen across the service over the same period).

Overall, we found no evidence of significant psychological or behavioral health effects attributable to the DTC among airmen who attended the program. Because we used a large sample and doubly robust methods to estimate the treatment effect, the effects were estimated with high precision. The findings rule out with relatively high confidence clinically meaningful improvement in mental health symptoms caused by the DTC. In contrast, while the study did not find a statistically significant causal effect of DTC attendance on binge drinking (even at a relaxed criteria of $p < 0.10$), the confidence intervals on the effect did not rule out the possibility of a clinically meaningful benefit.

Recommendations

The primary findings from this evaluation are that (1) one of the DTC program elements, as implemented, appears to be similar to posttraumatic debriefing interventions, which have been found to be either ineffective or harmful across several studies and are contraindicated by DoD, U.S. Department of Veterans Affairs, and World Health Organization clinical practice guidelines; (2) most program attendees believe that attending the DTC was a worthwhile experience that helped prepared them for reintegration; but (3) we did not observe benefits of DTC attendance on behavioral health or social conflict outcomes when attendees were compared with a matched group of airmen who did not attend the DTC. These findings are tempered by the limitations of the research design and available data. In particular, the studies that have evaluated posttraumatic debriefing interventions have been conducted primarily following noncombat trauma exposure in civilian populations. In addition, the findings of the quantitative assessment of the DTC are limited to the handful of measures that are available on the PDHRA assessment, which may not capture the full range of potential DTC outcomes.

Our recommendations depend largely on whether the outcomes included in this quantitative evaluation are deemed a good or poor match for the program's goals. If program administrators and Air Force decisionmakers view reductions in post-deployment PTSD symptoms, depression symptoms, binge drinking, and social conflict as constituting the core of the DTC's mission, then we would recommend that the resources directed to the DTC be invested in alternative programs or treatments that have been demonstrated to improve those outcomes. Specifically, we would recommend that the Air Force:

- Discontinue the DTC in its current form, and do not recreate the DTC for future conflicts using the existing procedures and programming; this program did not significantly reduce PTSD symptoms, depression symptoms, binge drinking, or social conflict following trauma exposure.
- Instead, invest resources in programs that have been demonstrated to reduce post-deployment PTSD symptoms, depression symptoms, binge drinking, or social conflict; or invest those resources into new, promising programs that the Air Force evaluates for beneficial effects.

On the other hand, if program administrators and Air Force decisionmakers decide that the outcomes assessed in this study are *not* the primary program goals, then our recommendations are quite different. For example, if the DTC is justified on the basis of goals related to R&R for airmen, or the collection of after-action information, the DTC may be a valuable program for the Air Force even in the absence of effects on behavioral health. In that case, we suggest that the Air Force:

- Revisit, document, and evaluate selected DTC program goals.
  - Develop a revised concept of operations that identifies how the program design, staffing, eligibility, and location are structured to achieve the goals that have been identified. For example, if R&R are key goals, the program materials should explain how the design, staffing, eligibility, and facilities relate to that goal. This may suggest changes to the DTC program.
  - Consider removing curriculum elements that have unsuccessfully targeted mental health goals, if such goals are not the primary focus of the program.
  - Develop an evaluation plan to empirically assess the effect of DTC attendance on important program objectives.
- Even if improving behavioral health is identified as a key program goal, remove the contraindicated program element of group processing of psychological trauma, and develop policy to prevent its reintroduction.

During our visit to the DTC, it was clear that the program staff were enthusiastic and committed to their mission. Participating airmen consistently noted the quality of the staff and the skill with which they approached their mission on satisfaction surveys. Unfortunately, many well-intended and well-liked programs prove to be ineffective. In many ways, the history of mental health prevention efforts could be summarized in the same way. It has proved extraordinarily challenging to reach the right people, at the right time, and with the right intervention to prevent the negative consequences of trauma exposure. In light of these challenges, it is not surprising that few prevention programs have been found to have benefits on post-deployment PTSD, depression, binge drinking, and social conflict. However, these evaluations are key for promoting ongoing program modification or program development that can improve outcomes for those airmen who serve their country on difficult or dangerous deployments.

Acknowledgments

We gratefully acknowledge the support of our current and previous project monitors at the Defense Centers of Excellence for Psychological Health and Traumatic Brain Injury, Yoni Tyberg, CAPT John Golden, and Col Christopher Robinson. We also acknowledge the support of many individuals at the Deployment Transition Center—in particular, Maj Lisa M. Hoyt. The quantitative evaluation of DTC effects would not have been possible without cooperation and data use agreements from the Armed Forces Health Surveillance Center (particularly Leslie Clark and Angelia Eick-Cost). We appreciate the comments provided by our reviewers, Mark Creamer and Gabriella Gonzalez. Their constructive critiques were addressed, as part of RAND's rigorous quality assurance process, to improve the quality of this report. We acknowledge the support and assistance of Lauren Skrabala, Christina Panis, and Barbara Hennessey in the preparation of this report.

CHAPTER ONE

Evaluation Approach and Program Description

Following the 1982 Falklands War, UK military personnel returned from the Falklands either entirely by sea or by sea to Ascension Island, where they transitioned to air travel (Hacker Hughes et al., 2008). For those who completed the entire journey by ship, travel time was one week longer. Popular press reports indicated that the psychological outcomes of those who traveled entirely by ship were better than those who returned home quickly, which was attributed to the time they had to decompress and debrief with comrades. Although formal outcome data to substantiate that claim have not surfaced, the narrative has entered into legend and is widely cited in support for providing decompression time between a war zone and home station (Hacker Hughes et al., 2008).

Indeed, with ready air travel, it is possible for service members to leave an active conflict zone and arrive home to be greeted by family within a matter of hours. There are possible disadvantages of such a system. Airmen who are exposed to significant risk of death in combat zone may benefit from decompression time before returning to their friends, families, and civilian settings. To exploit potential benefits of a decompression period prior to redeployment, in July 2010, the U.S. Air Force stood up the Deployment Transition Center (DTC) at Ramstein Air Base in Germany to provide airmen and Marines[1] redeploying (i.e., returning from deployment) from conflict zone deployments an opportunity to (1) *decompress* and (2) *share lessons learned* before returning to their home stations.

Evaluation Approach

Given the innovative nature of the program and potential for dissemination to other service branches, the Defense Centers for Excellence in Psychological Health and Traumatic Brain Injury contracted with RAND to complete an evaluation of the DTC that would:

- document and evaluate the structure and processes of the DTC program
- assess attendee satisfaction with the program
- evaluate post-deployment outcomes.

Our approach to achieving these aims included (1) a site visit, including interviews with DTC leadership and staff, (2) a review of DTC program materials, (3) a literature review of evaluations of interventions for individuals with trauma exposure, (4) review and summary

[1] Although the population served by the DTC includes a small number of Marines, we do not include Marines in the outcome analysis, and, for ease of reporting hereafter, we will refer to DTC participants as airmen.

of DTC-collected participant satisfaction data, and (5) an analysis of post-deployment outcomes as measured by the U.S. Department of Defense (DoD)-administered Post-Deployment Health Re-Assessment (PDHRA). All evaluation components were reviewed and approved by the RAND Human Subjects Protection Committee and received secondary approval from the Human Research Protections Office.

To document the structure and processes associated with the DTC, we visited the program site at Ramstein Air Base in Germany in September 2012. While there, we toured the facilities and interviewed program leadership and staff members. However, to protect the privacy of airmen attending the program, we did not meet with attendees or observe groups. We also reviewed DTC supporting materials, including the original concept of operations for the program when it was stood up and the 2014 revised concept of operations, which reflect the ways in which the program has evolved since it originally opened (U.S. Air Forces in Europe, 2014). We used the information gathered from the site visit, interviews, and DTC materials to document the structure and processes of the program. This report provides a description of the program as it was implemented at the time of our site visit.

To review benefits associated with the DTC and lessons for similar programs across DoD, we reviewed the literature on programs and interventions for individuals who have experienced a traumatic event that sought to prevent the development of lasting mental health problems. We used this review to identify programs that are similar to the DTC and to summarize their evidence base. We first reviewed the small but growing literature on third-location decompression (TLD) programs, which most closely match the DTC's program structure. Second, we reviewed the small body of research on non-TLD programs aimed at armed forces personnel. The selected programs included either debriefing or psychoeducational strategies to reduce the likelihood of mental health problems post-deployment. These programs did not include a rest and relaxation (R&R) component. Finally, we turned to the methodologically rigorous body of work on posttraumatic stress disorder (PTSD) prevention among civilians exposed to traumatic events. Although lessons from such programs may not be perfectly aligned with programs serving military populations, their outcomes provided a starting point for evaluation and helped to guide expectations regarding the DTC's outcomes.

To assess airmen's satisfaction with the program, we reviewed program participants' responses to a DTC-administered satisfaction survey. The survey contained four sections. The first queried attendees' opinions of the DTC overall, specific program content, and perceived skills and readiness to reintegrate with family and friends. The second section assessed respondents' current well-being, including perceived physical fitness, psychological well-being, and work-related quality of life. The third section included two questions about religious services, and the final section of the survey used open-ended questions to assess what each participant (1) liked about the DTC, (2) disliked about the DTC, and (3) would change about the DTC.

Finally, we assessed the differences between DTC attendees and a comparison group of similar airmen who did not attend the DTC. All outcomes were assessed using data available on the DoD-administered PDHRA questionnaire, given three to six months after return from deployment. We identified four measures on this assessment that map to DTC program goals: PTSD symptoms, depressive symptoms, binge drinking, and social conflicts with family and coworkers. Using individual participant identifiers and attendance dates for DTC attendees, we compared DTC attendees with a matched control group on the four available and relevant outcomes. Matching was done on the basis of airman and deployment characteristics that were assessed on the Post-Deployment Health Assessment (PDHA), a mandatory survey given within 30 days of the end of the deployment.

The purpose of this chapter is to provide a thorough description of the structure and processes of the DTC program as it was implemented in 2012. There are no publicly available resources that describe the program in depth, and such documentation can be valuable for the replication or dissemination of successful programs. Detailed program descriptions also provide the necessary background to enable selection of appropriate evaluation metrics. At noted above, the purpose of the DTC is to improve reintegration and behavioral health and social outcomes following deployments that involved exposure to adverse events. The program offered airmen an opportunity to (1) *decompress* and (2) *share lessons learned* before returning to their home stations.

Decompression

The DTC identifies "decompression" as a theoretical construct that promotes a healthy psychological response to deployment trauma. According to program materials, decompression has three elements: (1) *R&R*, (2) *debriefing* traumatic events experienced during the deployment, and (3) *preparing for reintegration* with family and friends. Most elements of the DTC, from logistical support to the formal curriculum for DTC groups, are intended to contribute to one or more of the decompression goals. Figure 1.1 shows the typical program schedule.

Rest and Relaxation

By design, service members who attend the DTC find that their travel and accommodation needs have been foreseen and arranged. DTC staff members arrange for weapons to be shipped to home stations and collaborate with travel representatives to book return air travel on commercial airlines. Except during periods of very high DTC utilization, participants are lodged

Figure 1.1
Schedule and Goals of DTC Groups and Activities

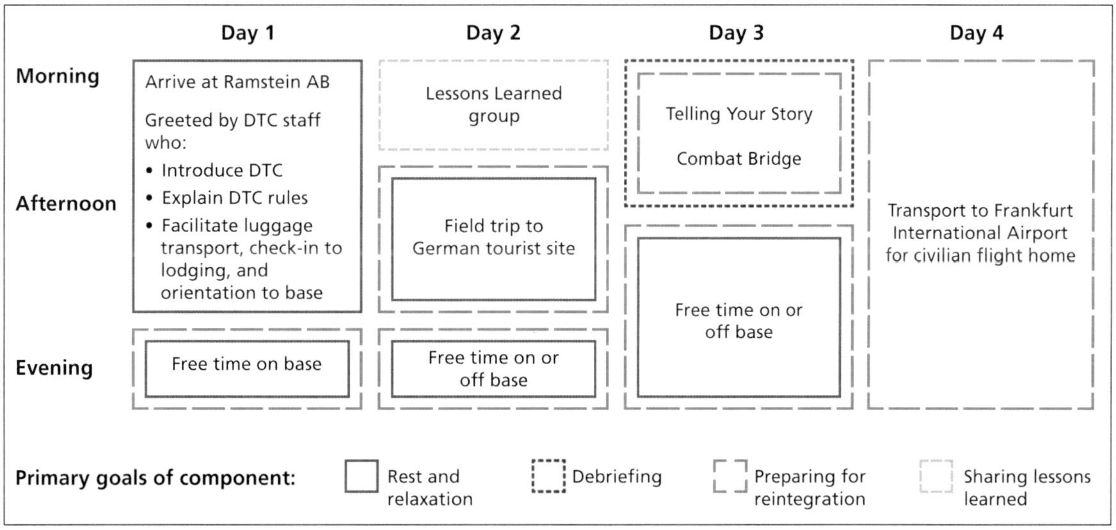

RAND *RR918-1.1*

on base, adjacent to the DTC program offices, in hotel-like rooms with a cleaning service. All bags are unloaded from the transport plane, transported to lodging by DTC staff, and left in each airman's room for their arrival. On arrival, airmen are given the schedule for their next two days at the DTC and the return flight information for their departure on the fourth day. All participants receive international phone cards to facilitate calls home to share with their families their precise arrival time. Ground transport is provided on base, and DTC staff members provide transportation to nearby German towns whenever possible. While attending the DTC, service members have access to wireless Internet service, computers, and the DTC operations center, which is staffed 24 hours and facilitates any needed services (e.g., transportation, pizza delivery). Whenever possible, morning start times for groups are scheduled late in the morning to allow adequate rest. In interviews, DTC staff members indicated that the goal of each of these seemingly small details is to remove as many of the inconveniences associated with deployment as possible to ensure that program participants can relax and recuperate.

The selection of Ramstein Air Base as the site for the DTC was motivated partially to contribute to the recuperation goal of the program. In interviews with staff members, they indicated that the "third location" setting (i.e., neither conflict zone nor home base) provides a neutral setting in which participants can focus on themselves without the stressors of a conflict zone or the demands of their family and friends. Ramstein was seen as a safe, peaceful setting in which to adjust slowly to the absence of conflict risks (combatants, improvised explosive devices [IEDs]), while readjusting to stimuli that may not have been present in the conflict zone (e.g., civilian vehicles, playgrounds, and nonthreatening crowds). The agricultural fields and mixed forests of southwestern Germany may also feel more familiar to many Americans than the climate and geography of Iraq or Afghanistan. Finally, a distant location maintains a significant geographic separation from family members and friends, which is seen as an important factor that allows service members to focus briefly on their own recuperation before returning to family.

In keeping with the R&R goal, DTC staff members also organize a half-day trip to a scenic German city on the first full day that airmen are on site. In some ways, this event is simply a field trip—a respite from a long deployment and an opportunity to see a German tourist site while passing through the country. However, much like many of the program components, it also provides an opportunity to adjust to a setting very different from their deployment. Walking the streets in civilian clothes without a goal or duty provides DTC attendees with a chance to practice skills that had once seemed commonplace: choosing a leisure activity, interacting with a restaurant server, paying for a purchase. It also provides an opportunity to note the behaviors that had been critical to life in a combat zone but that now must be phased out (e.g., constant vigilance, distrust of strangers, moving as a group).

Debriefing Significant Actions

On the morning of day 3 at the DTC, attendees gather in a DTC group room to discuss their experiences in the combat zone, a session that DTC staff members refer to as "Telling Your Story." Typically, groups are composed of 5–15 service members who were deployed together and are of similar ranks. The group leaders that we interviewed indicated that they start this session by asking about relatively innocuous events to "break the ice." Groups may be asked to share the funniest events that happened during their deployment or spend time talking about the events that defined the group. Group facilitators told us that the goal of this session is to eventually steer the group to discuss their worst or most traumatic significant action. In interviews with DTC staff members, they indicated that many groups, despite having gone through significant combat events, may never have discussed the event as a group. Staff members believe that it is important for groups who experience a traumatic event together to process that event together, which is thought to include the opportunity to hear the story from multiple perspectives.

Staff members do not encourage a particular emotional reaction to this debriefing but allow all reactions, whether neutral, angry, or sad. During our conversations with group leaders, we asked each whether there were any group processes that they specifically sought to avoid. No group facilitator volunteered that they avoided emotional recounting of trauma experiences. One staff members stated that they might call a short break during a session if they notice a group member becoming upset, but the opposite was more common, with some staff members indicating that emotional processing of the shared traumatic event or "catharsis" was an indication that the group was well run.

Preparing for Reintegration

Combat Bridge

Preparing for reintegration is addressed both formally and informally within the DTC structure. Formally, redeployers attend a psychoeducational group based loosely on the Army's post-deployment program Battlemind (Adler et al., 2009). Combat Bridge follows the Telling Your Story group on the third day and typically takes one to two hours to complete but may last as long as four hours. Group leaders continue groups until all components have been covered, rather than ending the session at a predetermined time. In these sessions, the group leader introduces four areas of functioning: physical, emotional/mental, social, and spiritual. For each area, the group completes a structured exercise in which they discuss the deployed environment and their coping strategies while downrange, followed by the extent to which each of these things would either remain the same or need to change when they returned home. For example, many of the physical conditions of a deployed versus a stateside environment are dramatically different, but in some cases, the physical coping mechanisms may be the same in both environments (e.g., "working out"). However, in many cases, coping mechanisms may need to shift on return to the home station. One of the goals of the Combat Bridge session is help service members rehearse new coping strategies that they can use (e.g., talking with a spouse) when old strategies are no longer available (e.g., hanging out with buddies).

Another goal of Combat Bridge is to prepare service members for the sometimes unforeseen stressors of reintegration. Although family reunions are almost always joyful, family reintegration can be challenging as the family readjusts to a long-absent spouse and/or parent, while the service member readjusts to the everyday demands of family life. When these challenges are predicted or expected, service members may be less likely to interpret them as a sign of failure or an indication that their relationships are faulty. During Combat Bridge, group leaders review service members' expectations for their return home and spend time discussing whether these expectations are (1) reasonable and (2) have been expressed to spouses, family, and friends.

Throughout Combat Bridge, group leaders review stress symptoms that are a normal part of reintegration (vigilance, sleep disturbances); the leaders also review resources that are available if these symptoms do not resolve within a few months post-deployment. Group leaders review Air Force and civilian resources for family reintegration and mental health support, seek to diffuse concerns about mental health stigma and confidentiality, and encourage airmen to seek help for themselves when necessary and to serve as advocates for fellow airmen who may be struggling with reintegration.

Informal Reintegration Support

Informally, the time at the DTC is designed to provide service members with a "pause" that allows them to adjust to the unfamiliarity of a civilian setting in order to be better prepared for reintegration when they do return home. It gives them a moment to remember the feel of civilian clothes and the security of a peaceful setting before they dive into the positive stressor of reintegration with their family and friends. DTC staff members work to note discrepancies between the setting and redeployers' behavior and to point out these discrepancies when they are noted. For example, when redeployers walk in formation through the streets of a German city, scanning the periphery, a DTC staff member will intercede to help them to recognize their behavior and adjust it to match their new environment. Finally, some of the program's policies (e.g., allowing limited alcohol use) are also designed to ease reintegration by providing scaffolding to help airmen slowly adjust to new freedoms.

Sharing Lessons Learned

The second goal of the DTC is quite distinct from the decompression goal and, rather than benefiting the individual service member directly, is designed to benefit the Air Force. On the morning of the second day at the DTC, service members attend a group to discuss the lessons learned during their deployment. The group leader discusses each component of the deployment, from notification to return. For each component, group members provide feedback about things that went well (e.g., pre-deployment trainings that were critical to success, indispensable equipment) and things that the Air Force could improve (e.g., missing uniforms, poor leadership). These groups are led by a recently deployed facilitator in the same career field as the group to ensure, among other things, that language and experiences are shared so that the discussions can focus on detailed lessons learned.

Following the Lessons Learned group, the group facilitator drafts an "after-action report" summarizing all feedback from group members. This report is forwarded to the Air Force career field chief at the Pentagon, who may use it to fine-tune the deployment process, training, or support of service members in the career field.

Although the primary product of the lessons learned group is the after-action report, DTC staff members believe that the group also has secondary benefits for redeployers. First, following a stressful and dangerous combat mission, it can be comforting to know that the hard-won knowledge gleaned from the deployment may be used to improve the experiences of other service members in the career field. Second, some DTC staff members see this group as a nonthreatening "warm-up" for Telling Your Story and Combat Bridge on day 3. Airmen may be suspicious of the mental health component of the program and reticent to engage in emotional processing of their experiences. The straightforward group experience associated with the Lessons Learned group, which is led by a group leader in the same career field, may help to remove their apprehension about the DTC.

Program Goals

The goal of the DTC is to provide airmen with the skills necessary to successfully reintegrate with their home station, workplace, and families (e.g., adaptive coping strategies, knowledge of military mental health resources). Designed and operated by Headquarters Air Force Services, the DTC is committed to preventing poor behavioral health outcomes among attendees. Based on a review of outcomes selected for an internal Air Force evaluation, briefings on the program, and our communication with program leaders, we identified reductions in post-deployment PTSD symptoms, depression symptoms, alcohol misuse, and social conflict as key program targets. Indeed, the DTC recruits a group of airmen who are at high risk for mental health problems and includes in its curriculum structured program elements that were originally designed for the purpose of reducing psychiatric symptoms or psychological distress following trauma exposure (Adler et al., 2009).

Despite these goals, in outward-facing materials, the program purposely avoids pointing to psychiatric outcomes as its primary target. There are a number of reasons that support this decision. First, the program is not intended or resourced to provide mental health *treatment* for those who have already developed psychiatric problems. Its purpose, instead, is to *prevent* currently healthy but trauma-exposed airmen from developing problems. Second, program goals are broad and include not only the prevention of psychiatric disorders, such as PTSD or major depressive disorder, but also subclinical anxiety and depression symptoms that do not rise to the level of a diagnosis but nonetheless have a negative effect on airmen's quality of life. Third, program developers recognized that stigma associated with psychiatric problems could serve as a barrier to airmen actively participating and benefiting from the program; if they were to perceive the program as a mental health program, they might choose to disengage.

Eligibility

Attendance at the DTC is limited to airmen who were regularly exposed to significant risk of death in direct combat or regularly exposed to traumatic events during their deployment. These experiences are associated with a high risk of psychological impact on airmen. The program has two routes to determine eligibility. At the time of this report, all members of four mission sets are preselected to attend the DTC: security forces, explosive ordinance disposal (EOD), tactical air control parties (TAC-P), and convoy operators. During the Operation Enduring Freedom (OEF) and Operation Iraqi Freedom (OIF) conflicts, these mission sets were identified as career fields that face regular exposure to risk of injury and death and likely exposure to significant actions and traumatic events. Airmen in these mission sets are prescheduled to attend the DTC following their deployment and may attend the DTC multiple times if they deploy more than once.

Eligibility may also be determined post hoc. Individuals or teams of airmen can be nominated by a deployed commander to attend the DTC if they were exposed to trauma. Specifically, each command-nominated individual must have experienced one of the following seven events: participated in direct combat operations, discharged weapon in combat, was injured in combat operations, was exposed to casualties or dead bodies, witnessed personnel killed or injured in combat, felt in great danger of being injured or killed, or experienced significant combat-related stress. DTC staff members estimate that approximately half of program participants are members of pre-identified mission sets, and half are command-nominated.

Staffing Structure

From the perspective of airmen who attend the DTC, their brief stop at Ramstein Air Base is a mix of a few processing and educational groups interspersed with time to relax and recuperate. Their seamless experience is carefully orchestrated and requires multiple levels of staff. The staffing structure is further complicated by dramatic variations in the number of attendees on site; on some days the DTC has no attendees, while at other times it serves several units of redeploying airmen. Because the redeployment schedule for units or airmen is determined by operational considerations in the field, rather than the DTC schedule, the DTC is constantly responding to changes in demand. DTC staff members anticipate and respond to these dramatic surges in demand so that all of the selected airmen can attend. To maintain flexibility, only a small number of staff members are permanent-party with two-year assignments. Many of the group leaders and logistic support persons are deployed to the DTC and, therefore, serve for only six months before returning to their permanent stations. These permanent-party and deployed staff are further supplemented by temporary duty assignments (TDYs), in which a potential group leader arrives at the DTC to complete a one-week training session and to lead one group before returning to a permanent station.

This staffing structure has some efficiencies, in that it allows for surges in simultaneous attendees without requiring a large number of permanent personnel, but is still very resource-intensive. In some cases, for example, TDY program staff may be flown to Germany for two weeks (including travel, training, and leading the groups) for the purpose of running six hours of small group discussions. A description of DTC permanent staff is included below.

The **DTC detachment commander** administers and oversees the DTC and is responsible for DTC staff and redeployers while they are participating in the program. Duties include implementation of the DTC mission, oversight of the annual operating budget, staff coordination, and liaison duties with deployed and home station commanders and support agencies.

The **DTC program manager** is an officer in a mental health career field[2] and is responsible for managing and training mission set managers and mental health technicians, overseeing the DTC curriculum, tracking program satisfaction among redeployers, reviewing the qualifications of potential group facilitators, and serving as the mental health consultant for attendees with significant mental health concerns.

The **DTC superintendent** (Senior Master Sergeant) coordinates manning requirements, local resources required to meet the mission, and professional development activities for DTC staff, and the superintendent addresses discipline issues as needed.

Group Facilitators

All DTC groups are facilitated by two leaders, one of whom is a colleague of the group members with a recent deployment within the same career field, and one of whom has some expertise in mental health (a mental health technician or chaplain). The Lessons Learned group is led primarily by a leader in the same career field (either the mission set manager or a career field

---

[2] At the time of our visit, the program manager was a licensed clinical social worker.

facilitator). The group leader with mental health experience is present for the Lessons Learned group and co-leads the discussion as necessary. On day 3, the roles switch. The Telling Your Story and Combat Bridge groups are led by the mental health facilitator, while the career field group leader co-leads the discussion as necessary.

Mission Set Manager

At the time of this report, the DTC served four primary mission sets: security forces, EOD, TAC-P, and convey operations. Each of these mission sets has a mission set manager (MSM), who is a senior airman (typically E-7) from the same career field with a recent deployment. MSMs sometimes co-lead groups of airmen in their career field or may assign a career field facilitator to do so. Their primary responsibilities are threefold. First, they are the liaison between the DTC and teams of airmen scheduled to redeploy. MSMs communicate with the leadership of deployed teams to learn about their combat experiences and group dynamics in order to design a DTC experience that will best meet their needs (e.g., breaking teams into appropriate groups, separating officers from enlisted service members). Second, MSMs are responsible for the final after-action reports for groups in their mission set and communicate with the Air Force career field chief at the Pentagon. Finally, MSMs are responsible for managing the career field facilitators who are deployed to the DTC and, when the deployed career field facilitators are inadequate to cover all expected DTC groups, for arranging TDYs for temporary group leaders. MSMs are deployed to the DTC and serve six-month assignments.

Career Field Facilitator

Career field facilitators (CFFs) are airmen with a recent deployment in the same career field as the redeploying airmen attending the DTC. They are responsible for co-leading DTC groups, taking primary responsibility for leading the Lessons Learned group and supporting the mental health leader during the Telling Your Story and Combat Bridge groups. CFFs' direct personal experience with the combat zone from which redeployers are returning is considered a critical component of the DTC program. Their real-world experience lends credibility to the DTC and helps to break down "us" versus "them" barriers between redeployers and DTC staff. CFFs are selected based on a supervisor's judgment that they have the aptitude for learning group management and basic counseling skills. However, they typically have no experience in a counseling role before their deployment to the DTC. CFFs are deployed to the DTC for six-month assignments.

Mental Health Technicians and Chaplains

At the time of our site visit, all mental health staff were mental health technicians or part of the chaplaincy. Mental health technicians take primary responsibility for the Telling Your Story and Combat Bridge groups and co-lead the Lessons Learned group. Mental health technicians also help provide training in group management and motivational interviewing to all newly deployed MSMs and CFFs, newly assigned mental health technicians, chaplains and chaplain assistants, and all TDY temporary group leaders. Mental health technicians also have a significant role in maintaining and updating the DTC curricula. Finally, although the DTC is not tasked with assessing mental health needs or providing mental health services, if it becomes clear that a group member has significant mental health concerns, the mental health technicians may triage the group member, consult with the program manager, provide appropriate referrals, and/or schedule an intake appointment with a mental health provider at their home base. Mental health technicians are permanent-party and assigned to the DTC for a two-year assignment.

Chaplains and chaplain assistants play a similar role as the mental health technicians, substituting for a mental health technician in leading these groups. Chaplains are also available to consult individually with redeployers if requested. Finally, they fill the unique role of ensuring that the spiritual needs of redeployers are met and that spirituality is included in the DTC curriculum. Chaplains and chaplain assistants are typically assigned to Ramstein Air Base and then complete a six-month assignment with the DTC.

Logistics

Staff support is also required to manage the significant logistics associated with the program. A **knowledge operations management journeyman** manages mail, computer hardware and software, and cell phones. A **services journeyman** coordinates air travel to and from Ramstein, schedules and maintains lodging facilities, and coordinates ground transportation. A **personnelist journeyman** in-processes and out-processes DTC staff and manages the arrival and departure of DTC redeployers. These positions are currently staffed by airmen serving six-month deployments.

Training Needs

Prior to arriving at the DTC, most MSMs and CFFs have no experience leading psychoeducational groups in active listening or in motivational interviewing. Mental health technicians and chaplains may have experience with group treatments or support groups. However, because the DTC is a unique program in the Air Force, no one will arrive with a history of running groups at a decompression program. To teach group leaders the skills they will need to facilitate DTC groups, experienced DTC mental health technicians and MSMs train all newly arrived group facilitators over a four-day period. The training includes direct didactics and observation of a complete group cycle. Training new group facilitators is a significant, ongoing investment for two reasons. First, MSMs and CFFs constantly rotate through the DTC on six-month deployments. Second, when a command-nominated group is scheduled to arrive at the DTC and that group is not in one of the four predesignated career fields, the DTC arranges a TDY CFF to travel to Ramstein for two weeks. That temporary CFF must be trained for four days prior to facilitating one DTC group, and then the CFF returns to his or her duty station.

Planning and Resources

Although the DTC necessarily delays homecoming, program staff are committed to minimizing that delay by serving airmen immediately after their deployment. That is, there are no wait times for program participation. Because the DTC has little control of redeployment dates and availability of air travel to Ramstein Air Base, this commitment presents a complex planning challenge. On some days, the DTC will have no airmen on site—meeting rooms and dormitories sit empty, and staff redirect their time to planning and preparation tasks. On other days, a 50-member team may arrive earlier than expected, stretching infrastructure and personnel availability to its limits and requiring additional TDY staff to meet demand.

Another key planning problem that the DTC had to solve was the commitment to ensuring that all redeploying airmen have a CFF with a recent deployment in the participants' career field. Given that commanders can nominate any group with an adverse event to attend the DTC—including those who only rarely attend the DTC—the MSM may need to quickly find, arrange a TDY, and train a recently deployed member of the career field to act as a group leader for a single DTC group. In any given time period, the DTC may be hosting airmen from the primary four career fields along with smaller groups from other career fields (e.g., medical officers). Thus, the planning task extends far beyond arranging for the arrival of the redeploying airmen.

Clearly, meeting the challenges associated with standing up and operating the DTC requires substantial infrastructure and personnel resources. The commitment the Air Force has made to the program suggests the strength with which leaders have valued and supported the mission of the DTC. Smoothing the transition from a challenging deployment back to the home station, providing an opportunity for R&R, and reducing the risk of poor behavioral health outcomes following trauma exposure during deployment are all important goals that the DTC has worked hard to meet. This evaluation seeks to determine the extent to which some of the goals have been met.

Summary

Recognizing the possible advantages of a gradual transition from a combat zone to the home station, particularly for airmen regularly exposed to traumatic events during their deployment, the DTC provides a brief pause between zones. During the two days of programming, the DTC gives airmen an opportunity to (1) decompress and (2) share lessons learned during their deployment. Decompression is a multifaceted process that includes rest and recuperation, a chance to debrief significant actions with the team who experienced them still intact, and, finally, a structured opportunity to plan for reintegration with family and friends. The program also includes an information-gathering component, the Lessons Learned group, which is designed to gather information about airmen's deployments to be passed back to the career field chief at the Pentagon. Although this component may have indirect benefits for redeployers, its primary goal is to improve future deployments. To support this multifaceted program, the management structure is supplemented with logistics and systems support and a variety of group facilitators each playing unique roles. Given the programmatic reliance on TDY and deployed staff, training needs are considerable and ongoing.

In the next chapter, we review the scientific literature evaluating programs similar to the DTC in structure, population served, or goals. A review of the outcomes associated with similar programs informed our expectations about plausible outcomes for the DTC.

CHAPTER TWO

Review of Reintegration and PTSD Prevention Programs

The DTC targets airmen who have been exposed to significant trauma events during their deployment and seeks to provide them with the decompression time, debriefing opportunities, and skills training that will help them to avoid the negative behavioral health outcomes that can follow trauma exposure. The DTC is not alone in these goals, and there are lessons to be learned from other programs that have targeted similar populations or sought to support resiliency in the face of negative life events. In this chapter, we review the scientific literature evaluating programs similar to the DTC in structure, population served, or goals. The results of this review helped to inform our expectations about the expected outcomes for the DTC.

Between 2001 and 2012, 2.5 million service members were deployed in support of OEF, OIF, or Operation New Dawn (Defense Manpower Data Center, 2013; U.S. Department of Veterans Affairs Office of Public Health and Environmental Hazards, 2010). In the era of the all-volunteer force, the pace and demands of these conflicts have resulted in longer and more frequent deployments and historically high levels of participation by reserve forces (Hacker Hughes et al., 2008; Deahl et al., 2000). Although most service members have coped well with deployment-related stresses, the high operational tempo of the past 14 years, longer deployments, and frequent redeployments have resulted in significant psychological health problems among service members.

PTSD, in particular, appears to be one of the most frequent psychiatric diagnoses among service members returning from OEF/OIF deployments (Schell and Marshall, 2008). Immediately following a deployment, 5–13 percent of service members screen positive for PTSD, and by six months post-deployment, these numbers have risen to 17–25 percent (Hoge, Auchterlonie, and Milliken, 2006; Milliken, Auchterlonie, and Hoge, 2007). In a large survey of OEF/OIF-deployed service members, 14 percent screened positive for PTSD, and, among these, nearly three-quarters screened positive for a comorbid condition, such as depression or traumatic brain injury (Schell and Marshall, 2008). Personnel who are injured or exposed to more extensive combat trauma are also at higher risk for developing PTSD compared with those without such experiences (Schell and Marshall, 2008).

In civilian settings, interventions for PTSD must necessarily occur *after* a traumatic event occurs. It is impossible to predict with precision who will be involved in a car accident, be sexually assaulted, or experience a natural disaster. Leaders in the military, however, are uniquely prepared to predict *a priori* who will experience a traumatic event. Those who deploy to a combat zone, and particularly those in high-risk career fields, such as EOD, are likely to witness or experience a traumatic event during their deployment. As such, multiple strategies to prevent and treat PTSD among military service members have been developed:

1. Before a deployment, resilience-based programming can be offered to prepare service members for traumatic events and train them to cope effectively in the face of such adverse circumstances. For example, Airman Resilience Training is a short, pre-deployment program designed to prepare airmen to cope with the day-to-day stress of a deployment and to react in a healthy and productive way if and when an adverse event does occur. Although this program has not fully lived up to its promise (Gonzalez et al., 2014), it is an example of a population-based prevention strategy designed to reduce the risk that airmen will develop mental health conditions following a deployment.
2. Alternatively, after a mental health condition has already developed, DoD can offer mental health services within the military health system. Multiple empirically supported treatments for PTSD are available (Benish, Imel, and Wampold, 2008; Bisson and Andrew, 2009; Bisson et al., 2007), and U.S. Department of Veterans Affairs (VA)/DoD clinical practice guidelines codify the provision of these services (e.g., the 2010 *VA/DoD Clinical Practice Guideline for Management of Post-Traumatic Stress*).
3. A third and less common approach is to identify airmen who have experienced an adverse event during their deployment and intervene with these airmen as soon as possible. This strategy seeks to identify those at highest risk for developing PTSD and provide targeted support in an effort to reduce the likelihood that they will develop a psychiatric condition. The DTC is one of the few programs that falls into this category.

We focus our review of the literature on programs that take the third approach—that is, programs that intervene with a population that has experienced a traumatic event in an effort to prevent the development of mental health problems. We use this review as a strategy to guide hypotheses about the value of a program such as the DTC by identifying similar programs and summarizing the evidence base supporting (or failing to support) those programs. We first review the small but growing literature on TLD programs. These programs match the DTC's program structure in their provision of debriefing and psychoeducational programming, their focus on R&R, and the selection of locations for the program that are distant from both the theater and the home station. Second, we review non-TLD programs aimed at armed forces personnel that include either debriefing or psychoeducational strategies to reduce the likelihood of mental health problems post-deployment but do not include an R&R component. This body of research is also small. Note that there are also a variety of reintegration programs supported by DoD. Many of these programs focus on civilian or military career reintegration outcomes (Werber et al., 2008, 2013, 2015), which are not the targeted outcomes of the DTC.

In situations in which a research literature remains underdeveloped, it is often helpful to turn to related research that matches the targeted intervention as closely as possible. Fortunately, there exists a methodologically rigorous body of work on prevention of posttraumatic psychopathology among civilians exposed to traumatic events. Supplementing the military-specific literature with research conducted with civilians has limitations and strengths. By definition, the population served and the providers implementing the program differ from the military population served by the DTC, which weakens our ability to generalize from their results. Nonetheless, the success or failure of these programs can provide a starting point for an evaluation and guide our expectations about the DTC's outcomes. In addition to reviewing programs for armed forces personnel, we also reviewed the three most widely disseminated programs for preventing PTSD among trauma-exposed civilians: psychological debriefing, psychological first aid, and trauma-focused cognitive behavioral therapy (TF-CBT).

Third-Location Decompression Programs

TLD programs are designed to help redeploying armed forces personnel transition from the "high-pressure" combat zone to the "low-pressure" home environment (Garber and Zamorski, 2012). They are physically located in a neutral zone that is neither the operational theater nor the individual's home station. Most programs include opportunities to debrief combat and other deployment experiences and offer psychoeducational programming to prepare the service member for the transition home. Notably, TLD programs also include a strong focus on R&R as an important strategy to assist the decompression process. Given this focus, countries that employ TLD programs for their service members often choose sites with high-quality lodging and ample recreational activities (tourist waterfront or sightseeing locations). Many allied countries—including Canada, the Netherlands, Australia, and the UK—support TLD programs for their service members. The priority for attendance is usually those personnel who may have experienced adverse events during deployment. The U.S. Air Force's DTC falls into this program category.

To our knowledge, a high-quality randomized controlled trial (RCT) of a TLD program has not yet been conducted. In the absence of such evidence, we turn to the available reports, which are limited to program implementation and participant satisfaction studies (Fertout, Jones, and Greenberg, 2012; Garber and Zamorski, 2012; Jones et al., 2011; Zamorski and Garber, 2013; Zamorski et al., 2012) and two propensity score–matching studies that evaluated the DTC (Schneider, Bezdjian, and Burchett, 2014; Roberts et al., 2010).

Surveys of UK service members who attended the British TLD program in Cypress reveal that service members are often reluctant to delay their homecomings by attending a TLD program (Jones et al., 2011; see also Fertout, Jones, and Greenberg, 2012). Forty-seven percent of participants indicated that they did not want to attend the program, and an additional 32 percent were ambivalent about attending. However, after completing the program, the majority of participants (91 percent) believed that the program was helpful. Even those who had not wished to attend were likely to report that the program was helpful (84 percent). The service members who were least likely to believe that the program was helpful were those in combat occupations, noncommissioned officers (NCOs), and those who had attended the program before (Mulligan et al., 2011a). Similar process evaluations with Canadian service members attending a TLD program also revealed initial ambivalence about attending the program followed by high levels of satisfaction (Garber and Zamorski, 2012; Zamorski et al., 2012), with support for TLD most strongly linked with service members' satisfaction with the education and R&R components of the program (Zamorski and Garber, 2013). Although participant perceptions of program helpfulness are important, these studies are unable to shed light on the outcomes associated with TLD. That is, they do not reveal whether program attendance improves positive coping and decreases negative outcomes after homecoming (e.g., alcohol misuse, PTSD symptoms).

Based on our review, the only outcome evaluations available on a TLD program were, in fact, prior evaluations of the DTC (Schneider, Bezdjian, and Burchett, 2014; Wirick, Garb, and Dickey, 2012). In January 2012, an unpublished report on the DTC was distributed (Wirick, Garb, and Dickey, 2012). In the report, the outcomes of airmen who attended the DTC in the first six months after it officially opened on July 1, 2010 ($N = 827$), were compared with the outcomes of a propensity-score matched sample of airmen who did not attend the DTC ($N = 13{,}679$). Six-month outcomes included routine screening questions from the PDHRA questionnaire, including the Primary Care PTSD Screen (PC-PTSD) (Prins et al., 2004); the AUDIT Alcohol Use Disorders Identification Test), a screener for problematic alcohol use (Babor and Grant, 1989; Bradley et al., 2003); and the Patient Health Questionnaire (PHQ-2), a screener for depression (Kroenke, Spitzer, and Williams, 2003). For the PC-PTSD, the recommended cutoff score for screening is endorsement of at least two of the four items (Prins et al., 2004). However the authors reported the percentage of airmen who endorsed at least one of the four items (Wirick, Garb, and Dickey, 2012). Fewer DTC participants endorsed at least one PTSD symptom (14.1 percent) than nonparticipants (23.4 percent; Wirick, Garb, and Dickey, 2012). It is important to note that a single symptom (e.g., nightmares) does not necessarily imply a diagnosable case of PTSD. Compared with the matched sample, airmen who attended the DTC had a similar likelihood of screening positive for depression but were less likely to screen positive for alcohol misuse at follow-up (27.5 versus 18.1 percent). In a review of medical record data collected during the six months following deployment, there was no evidence that DTC participants were less likely to be diagnosed with a mental health disorder compared with nonparticipants. However, consistent with the DTC focus on family and social reintegration post-deployment, a greater proportion of DTC participants (91.1 percent) relative to nonparticipants (84.4 percent) denied having serious family, social, or occupational conflicts. In sum, although the DTC had no effect on reducing the number of clinically diagnosable cases of mental health conditions post-deployment, there was some evidence to suggest that it may have improved reintegration outcomes (e.g., reduced alcohol misuse, improved family/social functioning). The Schneider, Bezdjian, and Burchett (2014) report contains a more complete methodological description and analyses than the brief, unpublished white paper by Wirick and colleagues. Given that Schneider and colleagues analyzed very similar data as our analyses, we summarize their findings and compare them directly to ours in Chapter Four and in greater detail in Appendix B.

It could be argued that the active component of TLD is simply time to decompress between a deployment and homecoming (rather than debriefing and psychoeducation opportunities). However, limited evidence suggests that the delay between leaving a deployment and returning home is not associated with health outcomes. An unpublished analysis conducted with the King's College cohort study of the physical and mental health of the UK armed forces capitalized on natural variation in time on base before being allowed on leave (reported in Hacker Hughes et al., 2008). Of 4,023 UK personnel returning from an operation in Iraq, 39 percent were sent straight on leave, 29 percent stayed on base for one to six days, 21 percent stayed on base for one to two weeks, and 11 percent remained on base for longer than two weeks. After accounting for demographic differences associated with time on base, the natural variation in delay of homecoming was unassociated with subsequent health outcomes, which may suggest that delay alone does not account for possible positive outcomes associated with TLD programs.

Post-Deployment Debriefing and Mental Health Psychoeducation Programs

Components of TLD programs can be implemented without the expense of R&R at a third location. That is, redeploying service members may participate in debriefing sessions or receive psychoeducation about mental health symptoms and family reintegration on return to their home stations. The documented outcomes of these practices is limited and mixed, with some programs demonstrating positive outcomes for those with high combat exposure (Adler et al., 2009) and others failing to show a positive impact associated with the program (e.g., Deahl et al., 1994).

In a 2011 review of the literature, seven intervention studies were identified that assessed the value of programs designed to prevent psychological health problems in military personnel returning from a deployment (Mulligan et al., 2011a). These brief, one- to three-hour programs typically are offered to service members after they experience a potentially traumatic event or shortly after return to the home base following a combat deployment. Most are structured as either a military debriefing session, psychoeducation about potential mental health symptoms with instruction about where to seek help, or both. The majority of these programs showed no effect on future PTSD symptoms (Mulligan et al., 2011a); however, two studies by Adler and colleagues showed a positive effect of psychoeducation and military debriefing among U.S. soldiers who had high levels of combat exposure (Adler et al., 2008, 2009). General psychiatric morbidity was assessed in four of the seven studies, and two showed a positive effect of the intervention during at least one follow-up time point (Mulligan et al., 2011a).

Two of the identified studies assessed the effect of post-deployment psychological debriefing on alcohol use and reported conflicting findings. Results from a nonrandomized trial showed that, relative to a comparison group, alcohol misuse was lower among those who received psychological debriefing one year following the intervention (but not at three or six months post-intervention; Deahl et al., 2000). The authors of a cluster-randomized trial of psychological debriefing reported that peacekeepers who received a debriefing intervention had *higher* rates of alcohol misuse three to four months after the intervention relative to a comparison group, who received a stress education program (Adler et al., 2008).

One of the studies included in the review above is of particular relevance to an evaluation of the DTC. Adler and colleagues (2009) conducted an RCT of Battlemind debriefing and Battlemind training with Army soldiers. It is worth highlighting this particular study both because of its methodological rigor and because the DTC uses materials based on the Battlemind model for its Combat Bridge session during day 3 of the program. The evaluation tested the effects of several brief, early interventions provided to returning soldiers in their first week after their return from an OIF deployment (Adler et al., 2009). Platoons were randomly assigned to attend one of three courses:

1. A standard stress education course developed by the Army.
2. "Battlemind Debriefing," a small group, military-style debriefing in which soldiers reflect on their deployment experiences and discuss the transition from combat to home. Battlemind group leaders are explicitly trained to avoid detailed, emotional recapping of trauma events (Adler et al., 2009). Positive coping strategies were discussed.
3. "Battlemind Training," a structured slide presentation reviewing normal responses post-deployment, mental health symptoms, and positive coping behaviors.

This evaluation showed that, relative to the typical stress education course, soldiers who attended Battlemind Debriefing or Battlemind Training had fewer PTSD, depression, and sleep symptoms four months after the intervention (Adler et al., 2009), but these reductions were true only among those who had high levels of combat exposure (Adler et al., 2009). Moreover, the effect size, even among those with high combat exposure, was small. For example, at follow-up, soldiers in the Battlemind debriefing scored three points lower on the PTSD

Checklist (Weathers et al., 1993) than soldiers in the standard stress reduction group. A three-point drop on in this scale score is not considered a clinically significant change (Monson et al., 2008; National Center for PTSD, 2012). In addition, it is not clear whether DTC participants have high levels of combat exposure as defined in the 2009 Adler and colleagues evaluation. While DTC participants are selected primarily based on the likelihood that they were exposed to trauma during their deployment, their average level of trauma may be lower than that of soldiers known to have high levels of combat exposure.

A replication of Battlemind training, adapted for British Armed Forces, was evaluated in a cluster RCT (Mulligan et al., 2011a). It differed from the Battlemind trainings conducted with American troops (reviewed above) in that it was implemented during a TLD program (similar to the DTC model), with platoons randomly assigned to receive either Battlemind training or the standard post-deployment brief. The evaluation showed a limited influence of the program at the six-month follow-up. There was no relationship between receipt of the UK version of Battlemind and mental health symptoms. However, there was a small reduction in binge drinking among program participants.

If the results of these Battlemind evaluations (Adler et al., 2009; Mulligan et al., 2011b) were to generalize to the DTC components similar to Battlemind training, we should expect the DTC program either to have no effect on mental health symptoms or to have a small effect on mental health symptoms. This generalization, of course, assumes that the DTC has no other active and effective clinical components beyond the Battlemind-like components—an argument that is difficult to support without further information.

Civilian PTSD Prevention Programs

Most TLD programs have operated only a short while—standing up during the OEF/OIF conflicts around 2005 (Garber and Zamorski, 2012; Hacker Hughes et al., 2008). At the time of this report, there are few studies on which to draw conclusions about their outcomes, and the evidence is mixed as to their influence on service members' reintegration experiences. In situations in which the literature remains underdeveloped, it is often helpful to turn to well-developed research programs that are as closely aligned with the topic of interest as possible. Fortunately, there exists a large body of research on PTSD prevention for civilians exposed to trauma.[1] These programs rely on prevention strategies similar to those implemented by the DTC and can help to guide hypotheses about the likely effects of the DTC.

Below, we review the outcomes of civilian PTSD prevention programs that either share commonalities with the DTC or have been demonstrated to be effective in some population: (1) psychological debriefing, (2) psychological first aid, and (3) TF-CBT. We use the conclusions of each research area to guide preliminary hypotheses about the likely outcomes of the DTC. We acknowledge that the civilian samples used in these studies differ in significant and substantial ways from the airmen who attend the DTC, and, therefore, the hypotheses are just that—best guesses based on the evidence already accumulated on a given approach to preven-

[1] We reviewed the literature on programs designed to prevent posttraumatic psychopathology, but we did not review the broader literature on psychological resilience or mental health promotion. However, the DTC may well also have effects on these outcomes. Thus, we include in our evaluation measures assessments of depressive symptoms and alcohol misuse.

tion. Ultimately, the analyses of DTC outcomes in the chapters that follow will be the best indicator of effectiveness of the DTC.

Psychological Debriefing

Psychological debriefing is a one-session, three- to four-hour intervention that targets trauma-exposed individuals, within two weeks of the trauma and preferably as soon after as possible (McNally, Bryant, and Ehlers, 2003). Group sessions are conducted with people who have been exposed to the same or similar traumas (e.g., the 9/11 attack on the World Trade Center), but may not have known one another prior to the event. Goals include the reduction of psychological distress and prevention of PTSD. In this approach, providers encourage group members to describe and relive the trauma in detail, with the expectation that emotional catharsis or ventilation will prevent development of more severe trauma symptomatology. These programs may be described as crisis intervention, psychological debriefing, critical incident stress debriefing (CISD), or traumatic event debriefing. A review of high-quality, randomized, and quasi-randomized trials concluded that debriefing does *not* prevent PTSD (Rose et al., 2002; see also McNally, Bryant, and Ehlers, 2003). Individuals exposed to a trauma who received a debriefing intervention were just as likely to develop PTSD as individuals who received either no intervention or an educational intervention. In fact, two studies reported that debriefing was associated with an *increased* risk of PTSD (Bisson et al., 1997; Hobbs et al., 1996). At this date, the recommendation in the scientific literature is not to conduct such interventions (McNally, Bryant, and Ehlers, 2003; Nash and Watson, 2011; Rose et al., 2002). As a result of a series of methodologically rigorous studies finding either no effect or adverse effects, current clinical practice guidelines for treating traumatized persons strongly suggest that such programs should not be used. This includes guidelines issued by the World Health Organization (World Health Organization Mental Health Gap Action Programme, 2012) and the *VA/DoD Clinical Practice Guideline for Management of Post-Traumatic Stress.*

The motivation to provide support to trauma survivors in the immediate aftermath of an extremely difficult event is empathetic and understandable. However, most survivors of a trauma demonstrate remarkable resilience, undergoing a natural course of recovery over several months that returns many people to their natural baseline (Rothbaum et al., 1992). During this period, survivors fluctuate between avoidance of thoughts and reminders of the event and engagement and processing of the event (Horowitz, 1986; Pennebaker and Harber, 1993). Some have argued that these early periods of avoidance allow survivors to focus their attention on the practical and necessary steps to rebuilding (e.g., finding new housing, completing medical treatments) and also provide time for the emotional intensity of their memories to fade (McNally, Bryant, and Ehlers, 2003). It may be that the emotional processing demanded by psychological debriefing is mismatched with the natural course of recovery. By forcing a particular type of processing at a particular time, the natural course of recovery may be disrupted by debriefing interventions. That is to say, some individuals who would have recovered on their own may now go on to develop posttraumatic psychopathology. Although systematic and emotional processing of traumatic events has been shown to be appropriate long after the event has passed (Powers et al., 2010), the empirical evidence does not support it in the immediate aftermath of a trauma (Rose et al., 2002) or in individuals who do not have significant symptoms of posttraumatic psychopathology. In fact, the *VA/DoD Clinical Practice Guideline for Management of Posttraumatic Stress* explicitly notes that debriefing is not recommended and indicate that "it is ineffective and may have adverse effects" (p. 107).

The DTC Telling Your Story group on day 3 of the program has some overlap with civilian-style psychological debriefing interventions. It appears that the DTC originally based this group on Battlemind Debriefing, a group debriefing for service members that explicitly trains providers to avoid emotional processing of the trauma event(s) (Adler et al., 2009). During site visit interviews, it appeared that some group facilitators did try to avoid emotional processing. For example, one group leader indicated that he or she would release the group for a short break if a group member was becoming upset. However, most facilitators interviewed valued "cathartic" group experiences and expressed support for emotional processing, with some suggesting that it was the hallmark of an effective group session. This latter approach to the Telling Your Story group shares similarities with the debriefing sessions that have been well studied among civilians and which are clearly contraindicated by the empirical literature (Rose et al., 2002).

During our interviews and review of training materials, we found no evidence that group leaders were directed to implement group emotional processing of traumatic events, but there was also no evidence that they had been cautioned against such strategies. This failure to explicitly train paraprofessionals to avoid debriefing-style prevention strategies is problematic. Without direction from leaders who are familiar with the empirical literature, it is not unreasonable to expect that group leaders will shift toward emotional processing of trauma events. Paraprofessionals have often been exposed to the evidence-based strategies with which to *treat* PTSD, which include exposure-based interventions that ask patients to recount their trauma events (U.S. Department of Veterans Affairs and U.S. Department of Defense, 2010). Without explicit guidance to the contrary, group leaders are likely to assume that treatments for people who *have* PTSD might also be helpful for people who are *at risk* for PTSD. Unfortunately, this logic does not match the scientific literature and may put attendees at risk.

If the DTC group mapped perfectly to civilian-style debriefing, we would predict null or harmful outcomes for the program. Of course, it does not map perfectly. Unique features of the DTC that distinguish it from civilian-style psychological debriefing make it difficult to use the poor outcomes of civilian groups to predict the likely outcome of the DTC. These differences include longer time delays between the adverse event and the Telling Your Story group,[2] the fact that group members are comrades rather than mere acquaintances or strangers, shorter group duration, and military cultural norms that may increase the likelihood that members maintain emotional composure during the group.

Psychological First Aid

In light of evidence that psychological debriefing interventions are either ineffective or harmful and guideline recommendations that caution against use of these strategies, providers who care for individuals in the immediate aftermath of a trauma have begun to look for alternative models of care. A model that is increasingly highlighted in the literature and in guidelines is psychological first aid (U.S. Department of Veterans Affairs and U.S. Department of Defense, 2010).

---

[2] Most participants will be describing an event that occurred more than two weeks prior to the DTC group. Of course, a few participants may have experienced their worst event just prior to redeploying and would therefore be processing the event on a timeline more closely aligned with civilian-style psychological debriefing. We expect that this brief delay between event and processing group would be the exception rather than the rule.

Psychological first aid is a modular, survivor-centered approach to the provision of services following a traumatic event. Services are matched to each individual and may be comprehensive for those who have limited resources and are coping poorly or may be minimal for those who are coping well (Brymer et al., 2006). The intervention seeks to deliver immediate posttrauma services that fill the following three needs:

1. Protection: Create a real or symbolic safe place and limit exposure to additional traumatic stimuli.
2. Direction: Direct survivors away from the traumatic site, severely injured survivors, and continuing danger.
3. Connection: Begin to reconnect the survivor with shared positive social values by choosing supportive and compassionate responses to the survivor and by providing practical assistance to reconnect them with loved ones, appropriate resources, and unit comrades.

The core objectives of psychological first aid providers are to engage the individual, provide safety and comfort, emotionally stabilize distraught survivors, identify the survivor's immediate needs, offer practical assistance to meet those needs, connect the survivor with social supports, provide psychoeducation about normal reactions to trauma and strategies to promote resilience, and, finally, provide information and contact information for services that may be useful in the future (Brymer et al., 2006). This list of objectives is not a one-size-fits-all intervention that is applied to every trauma survivor, and psychological first aid is not provided in group settings. Rather, the provider works with the survivor to deliver only needed and wanted care. Although psychological first aid manuals support ventilation of feelings and telling of the trauma story, this is recommended only when the survivor is motivated to do so (Litz et al., 2002). That is, providers listen and provide support to those survivors who choose to disclose their experiences, but never probe for details. The underlying principle of psychological first aid is to respect the individual's choices.

Psychological first aid has been described as "evidence-informed" (Hobfoll et al., 2007; Nash and Watson, 2011; Uhernik and Husson, 2009), a descriptor that indicates that elements of the intervention (e.g., positive social support) are supported by empirical evidence. For example, psychological first aid incorporates efforts to reconnect survivors with their social support network, which is supported by correlational evidence that shows that trauma survivors cope better when they have access to positive social support (Brewin, Andrews and Valentine, 2000; Ozer et al., 2003). However, the intervention itself has not yet been tested as a package to determine its effectiveness. As such, psychological first aid should be considered an experimental intervention with unknown treatment benefits and harms.

Psychological first aid differs substantially from the DTC approach to trauma survivors. First, it is a recommended approach immediately following the trauma (U.S. Department of Veterans Affairs and U.S. Department of Defense, 2010), whereas DTC attendance typically occurs weeks or months after the trauma (following the completion of the deployment). Second, psychological first aid is individualized, with each survivor receiving a unique "package" of services. Airmen who attend the DTC are not individually assessed to determine whether the DTC is well-matched to their needs, and upon arrival to the DTC, they attend the same series of groups and outings as all attendees. While there is variation in the degree to which attendees engage during group sessions, group leaders note that they call on nonparticipants to solicit their participation. Given that psychological first aid has not been evaluated, and that the targeted time frame for intervention is quite different than the DTC's, there are few inferences to be drawn from the literature on psychological first aid to predict the likely outcomes of DTC participants.

Trauma-Focused Cognitive Behavioral Therapy

An alternative to providing prevention services to all trauma-exposed individuals is to provide services only to those who have begun to develop traumatic stress symptoms (but who have not yet developed PTSD). This strategy depends on the ability to identify individuals with early trauma symptoms, such as acute stress disorder (American Psychiatric Association, 2013). Fortunately, simple, high-quality screening and assessment tools are readily available (Brewin, 2005), and screening for PTSD symptoms is already a standardized component of the PDHA completed by service members returning from a deployment.

The best-studied and most widely disseminated intervention for early trauma symptoms is TF-CBT, which is delivered only to individuals experiencing significant trauma symptoms and always within four weeks of the traumatic event. TF-CBT is a brief, four- to five-session therapy that includes education about stress responses to trauma, habituation to the trauma memory, real-world exposures to safe but avoided situations, and cognitive therapy to modify maladaptive beliefs associated with the trauma (U.S. Department of Veterans Affairs and U.S. Department of Defense, 2010; McNally, Bryant, and Ehlers, 2003). A systematic Cochrane review identified 12 high-quality studies that had evaluated TF-CBT for trauma-exposed individuals who had developed significant trauma symptoms and concluded that, compared with individuals who received either no intervention or supportive counseling only, individuals who received TF-CBT were less likely to develop PTSD (Roberts et al., 2010). In the 12 studies included in the systematic review, all participants had experienced a civilian trauma, such as a road traffic accident, physical or sexual assault, or occupational injury (Roberts et al., 2010). There are no known trials of TF-CBT among service members.

For military personnel with early signs of a stress reaction to a trauma, the *VA/DoD Clinical Practice Guideline for Management of Posttraumatic Stress* (2010) recommends TF-CBT. It is intended to be an individualized treatment that occurs in private sessions with a clinician and is delivered *only* to those experiencing stress symptoms. A trauma survivor whose natural course of recovery is proceeding smoothly should not receive this intervention.

The DTC approach shares some commonalities with TF-CBT. Like TF-CBT, Combat Bridge includes an educational component about common stress reactions to trauma and encourages positive interpretations of common reintegration problems (i.e., a behavior that was a positive skill in a combat zone must now be adapted post-deployment). Similar to the exposure component of TF-CBT, the DTC Telling Your Story sessions do include a retelling of the most significant adverse event. However, this session differs from exposure sessions, in which the patient retells the event *in the present tense* while attempting to recall all details of the event with strict fidelity. Moreover, exposure sessions are always repeated many times to ensure habitation, whereas the Telling Your Story occurs one time only, and habituation is not monitored. TF-CBT is delivered individually to those who have been identified with acute trauma symptoms, whereas DTC is delivered to a group of airmen without consideration of individual reactions to adverse events or individual need for the program. Although DTC participants may include some individuals experiencing acute stress reactions to a trauma that occurred within four weeks of the DTC stay (required for TF-CBT), most DTC participants will either be recovering well from an experienced trauma, will be separated from an experienced trauma by more than four weeks, or will not have experienced a significant trauma. Given the limited mapping of the DTC approach to the TF-CBT approach, we should use caution in generalizing the positive outcomes associated with TF-CBT to the DTC.

Summary and Predictions

Civilian PTSD programs—including psychological debriefing, psychological first aid, and TF-CBT—share some program elements in common with the DTC curriculum but lack true correspondence. Among other considerations, the DTC is a lengthy, multi-component, group-based prevention program. Even if we could be certain that correspondence was perfect between a civilian program (e.g., psychological debriefing) and a DTC component (e.g., Telling Your Story), it would still be inappropriate to use the null results associated with the civilian program to predict that the DTC will also be ineffective in preventing PTSD. Although one program element (e.g., Telling Your Story) is similar to interventions that have repeatedly shown no benefit, other program elements may exert opposite pressure to produce an overall positive outcome. Given these problems, we have based our predictions below on results from the evaluations that most closely match the DTC: a program evaluation of the first six months of DTC services and evaluations of Battlemind, a post-deployment curriculum that the DTC draws upon for its own programming (Telling Your Story and Combat Bridge).

Based on prior evaluations of the DTC (Schneider et al., 2014) and the Battlemind curriculum (Adler et al., 2009; Mulligan et al., 2011b), we expect that six months post-deployment, compared with matched nonparticipants, DTC program participants will

1. have PTSD, depression, and alcohol misuse scores that are statistically lower but that are clinically insignificant in size
2. be less likely to report significant conflict with family members, friends, or coworkers.

In closing, we note that the DTC does not define itself narrowly as a prevention program for psychiatric diagnoses, but rather sees its mission more holistically as a strategy to improve post-deployment mental and behavioral health across a full spectrum of functioning following a stressful deployment to a combat zone. Although an evaluation that showed that mental health outcomes improved following exposure to the DTC would be welcomed,[3] program leadership also see other potential benefits of the program. For example, if it were determined that the "only" benefit of the program is to provide redeploying airmen a deserved opportunity to rest and relax before rejoining their families and home stations and to instill the knowledge that stress reactions are normal, shared, and solvable, we believe that leadership may perceive the program as a success.

[3] Indeed, unpublished results from the prior evaluation of DTC suggesting program benefits on psychiatric symptoms have been widely circulated by DTC staff as part of their briefings about the program.

CHAPTER THREE

Participant Satisfaction with the Deployment Transition Center

Introduction

Attendees had the opportunity to describe their experiences at the DTC through a satisfaction survey, which was administered to airmen at the end of their stay. In this chapter, we present the results of this survey, including quantitative ratings and qualitative descriptions of several notable aspects of the program.

Methods

Survey Structure and Content

Airmen completed surveys at the end of their DTC stay (day 3; see Chapter One), following all scheduled activities except "check-out" operations, which were scheduled for the next day (day 4). According to DTC program staff, surveys were administered privately on a computer and completed between May 2012 and April 2013. A total of 1,552 airmen submitted surveys. Data on the number of airmen invited to complete surveys were not collected, so a precise response rate is unavailable, but it appears to be a substantial majority of those who attended over those dates.

The DTC satisfaction survey contained four separate sections. The first section (14 items) queried attendees' opinions of the DTC overall, specific program content, and attendees' perceived skills and readiness to reintegrate with family and friends. Items had the following five response options: strongly disagree, disagree, neutral, agree, and strongly agree.

The second section (15 items) covered respondents' current well-being, including perceived physical fitness, psychological well-being, and work-related quality of life. These items had five response options: very low, low, average, high, and very high.

Two questions about religious services comprised the third section of the survey. The first item addressed attendees' perceptions of their ability to attend a worship service given the DTC schedule. Response options were not at all, rarely, sometimes, usually, and any time I wanted. The second item addressed actual attendance of a worship service at the DTC. Response options for this item were: no, I did not wish to attend; no, but I wanted to go; once; twice; and each time there was a service available.

The last section of the survey included three open-field items for respondents to describe:

1. what they liked about the DTC
2. what they disliked about the DTC
3. what they would change about the DTC.

Qualitative Data Coding Procedures and Analysis

Two coders iteratively derived a set of codes based on responses to all three open-field items (what did you like/dislike/want to change about the DTC). Codes for each item were mutually exclusive. Cross-field codes included *structural* elements of the program (e.g., location, accommodations, duration, requirement to attend, and environment), program *processes* (e.g., class format and content, logistics, rules and regulations, and personnel), and intermediate (or proximal) *outcomes* (e.g., attendees' perceived ability to meet the goals of the DTC; Donabedian, 1966, 1980). Because surveys were administered while attendees were at the DTC, no long-term outcomes (e.g., actual success at reintegration) were assessed.

The coders independently coded a random sample of 5 percent of the data, and consensus was met regarding the codebook. The updated codebook guided their coding of a second random sample of 5 percent. Finally, one coder coded the remaining 90 percent of items, and the second coder double-coded 10 percent of those; inter-rater agreement was high. Coding disagreements were resolved through consensus. Overall, 20 percent of the responses were double-coded to ensure the reliability of the coding system.

Survey Data Limitations

The results of the DTC satisfaction survey should be considered within the limitations of the data available. Specifically, the survey was designed, fielded, and tabulated by DTC program staff, and we cannot describe those research methods. These data were provided to RAND in aggregate form. As such, we were unable to determine whether outcomes were associated with individual characteristics, such as gender, rank, or deployment experience. It also precluded us from analyzing changes in individuals' outcomes from before to after the DTC. Relatedly, DTC did not collect outcomes for a control group (i.e., individuals who were DTC-eligible but who did not attend the DTC); as such, we could not determine—via these surveys—whether DTC attendees were systematically different from other similar redeployers. As such, the data presented below are descriptive, providing a general picture of airmen's experiences at the DTC and their general subjective states as they left the DTC and prepared to return home.

Results

Overall Satisfaction with the DTC

The majority of DTC attendees reported that the DTC was a worthwhile experience (80 percent agreed or strongly agreed), and that it helped to prepare them to return home (74 percent; Table 3.1). In general, attendees reported that the general DTC concept, including having a time to rest (76 percent) and decompress (83 percent), as well as formal instruction about how to reintegrate after deployment (78 percent), was good. Although, on average, satisfaction was high, a sizable minority of airmen was ambivalent about or dissatisfied with the program.

These sentiments were also generally reflected in the qualitative responses from attendees, who were likely to offer comments on their overall DTC experience: Among the 339 participants who commented on their overall satisfaction with the program, 92 percent reported liking the DTC. For example, one respondent wrote, "It was a wonderful experience for me. I liked the whole program." Participants who commented also often noted liking the ability to relax and having the opportunity to talk. For example, in response to the question about what they liked about the DTC, one respondent wrote, "A chance to relax before going home. . . .

Table 3.1
Overall Satisfaction with the DTC

Category	Statement	Strongly Disagree % (*n*)	Disagree % (*n*)	Neutral % (*n*)	Agree % (*n*)	Strongly Agree % (*n*)
Overall	Overall, the DTC was a worthwhile experience	3.5% (49)	4.8% (68)	11.6% (164)	38.8% (548)	41.3% (584)
	The DTC experience was beneficial to my fellow unit members preparing to return home	2.3% (33)	3.0% (42)	20.9% (295)	43.6% (616)	30.2% (427)
DTC concept	It was helpful to have the DTC to rest and decompress before going home to family/friends	4.2% (60)	5.7% (81)	13.9% (197)	35.2% (497)	40.9% (578)
	I think decompressing and letting off steam before returning home is a good idea	2.9% (41)	2.3% (32)	12.0% (169)	36.4% (515)	46.4% (656)
	It was helpful to receive some guidance and recommendations to facilitate a smooth transition/reintegration with my family/friends	3.0% (42)	3.8% (54)	15.0% (212)	44.8% (633)	33.4% (472)

Also being able to talk about the experience with folks who know what you are experiencing versus judging." Of those who commented on their preparedness to return home, their comments were overwhelmingly positive. For instance, one respondent's comment that broadly represented the others was "I am more aware of my physical and mental needs when I deploy home. It was a great course, thank you!!"

Structure of the DTC

The DTC satisfaction survey did not include explicit questions about the structural elements of the program; however, many respondents commented on the structure of the program in the open-field portions of the survey (see comment codes in Table 3.2). Specifically, among those who commented on the DTC accommodations, 67 percent reported that they liked the DTC accommodations, particularly the rooms in which they stayed, noting that the generous accommodations contributed to the perceived effectiveness of the DTC. For example, one respondent wrote, "Comfortable living conditions greatly enhanced decompression." Similarly, among those who offered comments on the DTC environment, the vast majority (96 percent) described it as a relaxing, stress-free atmosphere. One participant wrote, "I loved the atmosphere, and the 'no-pressure' feeling I had during the duration of the course." On the other hand, among those offering comments on the DTC location, the tone of those comments was mixed. Respondents often commented positively (49 percent) about being in Germany and negatively (25 percent) about the distance between their living quarters and other buildings on the base, such as restaurants or the gym.

DTC Processes

DTC attendees rated their satisfaction with DTC program processes with questions from the structured portion of the survey (Table 3.3). In general, respondents rated the classroom modules highly, with approximately two-thirds or more agreeing or strongly agreeing that each module assessed was helpful and increased reintegration knowledge and skills. Similarly, the

Table 3.2
Comments on DTC Structure (Qualitative Codes)

Code	Total Comments (*N*)	Positive % (*n*)	Negative % (*n*)	Suggested a Change % (*n*)
Accommodations	273	66.7% (182)	14.3% (39)	19.0% (52)
Environment	160	96.3% (154)	2.5% (4)	1.3% (2)
Location	138	49.2% (68)	24.6% (34)	26.1% (36)

Table 3.3
DTC Processes (Quantitative Items)

Category	Statement	Strongly Disagree % (*n*)	Disagree % (*n*)	Neutral % (*n*)	Agree % (*n*)	Strongly Agree % (*n*)
Classroom activity	It was helpful for me to talk about my own deployment experiences	3.3% (47)	5.4% (76)	22.9% (324)	39.3% (555)	29.1% (411)
Classroom module	The "transition to home" training was helpful, and increased my reintegration knowledge and skills	3.1% (44)	4.5% (64)	18.7% (264)	44.0% (622)	29.7% (419)
	The "Tell Your Story" discussion was helpful and increased my reintegration knowledge and skills	3.8% (53)	5.6% (79)	22.2% (314)	40.2% (568)	28.2% (399)
Length	The DTC training was just the right length	4.0% (56)	6.4% (90)	17.9% (253)	41.9% (592)	29.9% (422)

majority indicated that the length of the DTC was "just right." However, there was a substantial minority of attendees (approximately one-quarter to one-third) who were either ambivalent about or dissatisfied with DTC content.

Analysis of qualitative data from open-ended questions provided additional insight into airmen's satisfaction with DTC processes (Table 3.4). Process-related themes that emerged in the qualitative data were classroom content and format, program format (e.g., schedule, activity type), various program rules and regulations, and aspects of implementation, such as logistics and personnel. These were coded as being positive comments, negative comments, or suggestions for change.

Classroom

Attendees were generally satisfied with the content and format of the classes. The small class size, the open discussion format, the relaxed classroom atmosphere, and the quality of the facilitators were all noted as well-liked aspects of the DTC. One respondent reflected generally on the class, writing, "The classes were pertinent, to the point, and allowed a lot of room for discussions that facilitate the decompression." Comments that addressed the open discussion format were common. For example, one respondent wrote, "Classes were informal and you were able to speak freely about your experience during deployment." Having facilitators who shared in the deployment experience was important for many respondents. For example, one

Table 3.4
DTC Processes (Qualitative Codes)

Category	Code	Total Comments (*N*)	Positive % (*n*)	Negative % (*n*)	Suggested a Change % (*n*)
Classroom	Class Content	104	57.7% (60)	28.8% (30)	13.5% (14)
	Class Format	165	60.6% (100)	21.8% (36)	17.6% (29)
Format	Duration of DTC	190	17.4% (33)	47.9% (91) (too short)	34.7% (66) (too long)
	Program Format	361	39.1% (141)	23.5% (85)	37.4% (135)
	Requirement to Attend	169	3.6% (6)	47.9% (81)	48.5% (82)
	Timing of DTC	19	10.5% (2)	63.2% (12)	26.3% (5)
	Talk	253	92.5% (234)	4.0% (10)	3.6% (9)
	Travel	361	65.4% (236)	4.4% (16)	30.2% (109)
Implementation	Logistics	337	30.0% (101)	34.4% (116)	35.6% (120)
	Personnel	342	90.9% (311)	5.6% (19)	3.5% (12)
Rules	Alcohol Rules	54	18.5% (10)	50% (27)	31.5% (17)
	Curfew Rules	68	1.5% (1)	63.2% (43)	35.3% (24)
	Other Rules and Regulations	127	42.5% (54)	36.2% (46)	21.3% (27)

wrote, "The class sessions were facilitated well. Having experienced staff and those that had 'been there, done that' made a difference."

Format

Many respondents commented on the duration of the DTC, but the results were mixed between liking the length, finding it too short, and finding it too long. For example, one participant wrote, "I would've liked to spend more time here to decompress." However, some participants felt that it was too long and were eager to get home: "Make it shorter. A lot of us just want to be home."

Those who commented on the requirement to attend the DTC overwhelmingly expressed dislike; almost half were in favor of changing the requirement. In particular, those who disliked the program did not like being kept from their homes for additional days. "The delay in returning me to my family was more stressful than just letting me go home and decompress with my wife, kids, and pets." Many participants recommended that the requirement to attend be made optional or be based on the deployment experience of each unit. For example, one respondent wrote, "If a unit does not receive contact—they should not have to attend this course. I learned nothing and did not benefit from this course. It was unnecessary."

Attendees frequently commented on the program format. Those who commented positively on the format enjoyed the balance of class time and free time. For example, one participant wrote, "I liked that we were not confined to a classroom the whole day and actually were allowed to be on our own and determine our schedule after the class sessions." Many also requested that the DTC provide optional one-on-one time with a counselor.

Implementation

Comments about logistics were also common and included positive and negative feedback, as well as several suggestions for change. Many of those who indicated that they were pleased with the logistics/organization commented that once on base, the organization of the program was great. One attendee wrote, "The setup is actually really great. They do an excellent job of billeting and squaring away arrival. Everything is pretty much taken care of for you." Many of the negative comments were related to the lack of adequate and reliable transportation on the base. One attendee wrote, "There was a complete lack of organized transportation. . . . Maybe a shuttle that runs hourly or every two hours would be beneficial." Attendees also expressed concern about the process of getting to the DTC and suggested that attendees receive information about the DTC before arriving, such as an itinerary and a map of the base.

DTC personnel were overwhelmingly well liked, including both the class instructors and logistics support staff. One attendee wrote, "Knowledge and expertise were second to none. First rate service and concern for each member." Another participant wrote, "I liked the fact that there was an instructor who had experienced the deployment process and understood the things that we went through."

Many attendees also mentioned the off-base sightseeing excursion, and among those who did, most were in favor. One praised "the opportunity to . . . see the beautiful countryside and reintegrate with society without the stressors of home." Those who suggested changes to the sightseeing portion of the program wanted to make the field trip optional.

Rules

The comments related to various rules and requirements were mixed. In general, those restricting behavior were disliked, and those enabling relaxed requirements were well liked. For example, regarding the limit on alcohol consumption, one respondent wrote, "I feel that putting limits on drinking and having a curfew was a bit much. We are adults, so please treat us as such." Others made positive comments about some of the relaxed requirements put in place, such as uniform rules. One wrote, "I liked that you could just go back to the civilian life style and not have to worry about rank or checking your uniform was not mess[ed] up."

Attendee Well-Being and Perceived Readiness to Reintegrate

Through the structured survey items, DTC attendees described their current well-being, including perceived physical health, emotional well-being, and work-related quality of life (Table 3.5). In general, respondents indicated that their well-being was good, noting positive perceptions of their physiological well-being (fitness and sleep) and that the DTC gave them the ability to relax. They reported high levels self-confidence, and reported their family stress, fear, sense of danger, and temper to be low. Work-related quality of life, including sense of

Table 3.5
Attendee Well-Being Post-DTC (Quantitative Items)

Category	Item	Very Low % (*n*)	Low % (*n*)	Average % (*n*)	High % (*n*)	Very High % (*n*)
Please rate the following items in terms of their current levels TODAY:						
Physiological well-being	Physical fitness	1.0% (14)	3.3% (46)	30.8% (432)	41.6% (584)	23.3% (327)
	Amount of sleep	0.9% (13)	8.3% (116)	40.1% (563)	34.4% (483)	16.3% (228)
	Quality of sleep	0.9% (12)	9.1% (127)	33.0% (463)	36.7% (515)	20.4% (286)
	Ability to relax/ decompress	1.4% (19)	3.3% (47)	38.1% (535)	35.4% (496)	21.8% (306)
Emotional well-being	Attention to detail	0.4% (5)	0.9% (13)	25.7% (361)	46.3% (649)	26.7% (375)
	Environmental awareness	0.6% (8)	1.1% (15)	27.9% (391)	42.6% (598)	27.9% (391)
	General fear	41.9% (588)	30.3% (425)	24.7% (347)	2.1% (29)	1.0% (14)
	Hot temper	33.1% (464)	28.4% (399)	29.6% (415)	7.9% (111)	1.0% (14)
	Level of family stress	28.7% (403)	27.7% (388)	34.1% (478)	7.9% (111)	1.6% (23)
	Self-confidence	0.3% (4)	0.8% (11)	22.0% (309)	46.0% (646)	30.9% (433)
	Sense of personal danger/threat	32.6% (457)	26.7% (374)	27.8% (390)	8.7% (122)	4.3% (60)
	Sense of personal safety	5.5% (77)	4.6% (65)	37.1% (521)	31.6% (444)	21.1% (296)
Work-related quality of life	Desire to separate from the Air Force	31.9% (448)	21.6% (303)	29.7% (417)	9.9% (139)	6.8% (96)
	Level of work stress	28.5% (400)	29.7% (416)	34.9% (490)	5.9% (83)	1.0% (14)
	Sense of pride in squad/team/unit	3.3% (47)	4.7% (66)	33.6% (471)	32.9% (461)	25.5% (358)

pride in the squad, was positively perceived by respondents. Work stress and desire to separate from the Air Force were low.

Airmen also described their readiness to return home in terms of their skill and emotional preparedness for reintegration (see Table 3.6). Overall, a large majority of airmen reported that they had the skills (>91 percent agreed or strongly agreed) and were emotionally prepared (87 percent agreed or strongly agreed) to reintegrate home.

Responses to the open-field items were consistent with the quantitative data described above. Specifically, among those who commented on their emotional readiness to return home, the vast majority described appreciating having time to spend alone (94 percent), relax (99 percent), and spend social or bonding time with their fellow airmen in a safe environment before

Table 3.6
Skills and Emotional Preparedness for Reintegration (Quantitative Items)

Category	Statement	Strongly Disagree % (*n*)	Disagree % (*n*)	Neutral % (*n*)	Agree % (*n*)	Strongly Agree % (*n*)
Skills	I have a good understanding of what I might expect during the process of transitioning back home and reintegrating with family/friends	0.8% (12)	0.6% (8)	7.4% (104)	52.6% (743)	38.6% (546)
	I know what I need to do if I need help with post-deployment reintegration issues	0.8% (11)	0.3% (4)	5.4% (76)	52.0% (735)	41.5% (587)
Emotional preparedness	I feel my fellow unit members are mentally/emotionally prepared to return and reintegrate	0.5% (7)	1.1% (16)	13.4% (189)	53.6% (757)	31.4% (444)
	I'm mentally/emotionally prepared to return home to my normal work duties and daily routine	0.5% (7)	1.0% (14)	11.0% (156)	52.7% (745)	34.7% (491)
	I was able to sleep, rest and restore my energy	1.9% (27)	3.3% (46)	15.0% (212)	42.2% (596)	37.7% (532)

returning home (95 percent; see Table 3.7). One participant summarized this concept, writing, "The most important aspect of the DTC is having downtime together with the people you deployed with before returning home. . . . [It] lets everyone relax and not feel anxious about getting home." They also liked that they had the skills that they felt they needed to reintegrate upon returning home (95 percent). Many respondents felt that the DTC allowed them to work through their thoughts and emotions, noting the opportunity "to fully evaluate our fears and stressors and plan for actions to overcome difficulties on returning home." For other participants, the preparation for home was more specific to their concerns. One wrote, "The DTC was an excellent way to prepare for the interaction with my family and friends. I was worried about how distanced my daughter might have become, but know now that it's normal and how to deal with that."

Table 3.7
Well-Being and Readiness to Reintegrate (Qualitative Codes)

Outcomes	Code	Total Comments (*N*)	Positive % (*n*)	Negative % (*n*)	Suggested a Change % (*n*)
Emotional	Alone	16	93.8% (15)	6.3% (1)	0% (0)
	Relax	293	99.3% (291)	0.3% (1)	0.3% (1)
	Social/Bonding Time	91	94.5% (86)	2.2% (2)	3.3% (3)
Skills	Prepared for Home	161	95.0% (153)	4.3% (7)	0.6% (1)

Summary

Data from quantitative and qualitative survey responses indicate that airmen were satisfied with their experience at the DTC. They especially liked the accommodations, being in Germany, and the balanced schedule, as well as the relaxed, stress-free environment and the opportunity to talk openly. Negative comments were generally in the areas of transportation; program rules, such as alcohol limits and curfew; and mandatory attendance at the DTC. There were numerous suggestions to improve the shuttle system. There were also suggestions to revisit the protocol for selecting DTC attendees, including making attendance optional or taking into consideration whether each airman saw combat during the deployment. Other suggestions included making the field trip optional and improving the logistics leading up to the DTC, such as having a better idea of what to expect at the DTC and what to bring.

In the future, DTC leaders may wish to include questions to test attendees' retention of the information conveyed in Combat Bridge. That is, the psychoeducational components of the program can be evaluated with tests similar to other educational evaluations. For example, it can be useful to assess not only whether attendees believe they are prepared to address mental health symptoms that may arise, but also whether they *remember* the contact offices that they can reach out to for help if necessary. It may also be useful to schedule a follow-up assessment with a sample of attendees to assess their satisfaction with the program and beliefs about their preparation for reintegration after they have actually been through the transition process. Post-reintegration perspectives on the program may be different than pre-integration perspectives and can provide useful information to program planners.

Overall, DTC attendees provided important information for the Air Force to consider when making structural-, procedural-, or outcome-related decisions about the DTC.

DTC attendees suggested that the following program elements continue:

- Maintain the high-quality accommodations already provided.
- Maintain the existing schedule that balances class time and free time and provides ample opportunity for attendees to just relax.
- Continue to recruit experienced and highly engaged personnel to staff the program.
- Maintain the highly organized, logistically sound processes of arrival to the DTC.
- Continue to provide the off-base sightseeing trip, but consider making it optional.

DTC attendees suggested reconsidering the following program elements:

- Revisit the protocol that determines who attends the DTC to ensure that it is available to those who need it most and not required for those who do not need it.
- Consider improving the transportation options for attendees while on base and to nearby offsite locations.
- Reconsider some of the restrictive DTC rules and requirements.
- Consider ongoing review of the preparation process leading up to the DTC, in addition to providing additional information about the DTC prior to attendees' arrival, to ensure that these processes run smoothly.

CHAPTER FOUR

The Effects of DTC Attendance on Psychological Symptoms, Alcohol Use, and Social Conflict: A Propensity Score–Based Approach

The gold standard in evaluating an intervention is the randomized controlled trial (RCT). In an RCT, individuals who are eligible for a treatment program are randomized either to a group that receives the treatment or to a control group that does not receive the treatment. The effect of treatment can then be estimated by examining the difference in average outcomes between the groups. Evaluating the DTC via RCT is not feasible; there is a commitment in the Air Force that all eligible airmen be served by the DTC rather than randomized into a group that may not receive treatment. Hence, there is a need to employ an alternative approach to estimate the effect of attending the DTC.

Propensity score analytic methods are designed to estimate a treatment effect that is similar to what would be found in an RCT, but can be estimated even when participants were not randomly assigned to treatment. The propensity score approach that we employ compares the treatment group (i.e., the group of airmen who attended the DTC) to a control group of airmen who are equivalent to the treatment group on all measured background variables, but who did not attend the DTC. That is to say, a comparison group of airmen whose career fields, trauma exposure, and deployment characteristics match the distributions of those who attended the DTC. Specifically, the primary analysis creates a control group of airmen who appear to be eligible to attend the DTC and who match the characteristics of those who did attend, but who could not attend because their deployment predated the opening of the DTC in July 2010. The analyses then compare DTC attendees with the matched control group on key outcomes, including PTSD symptoms, depression symptoms, alcohol use, and conflicts with family and coworkers. Outcomes were assessed following reintegration, several months after returning from deployment.

Methods

Data Sources

Staff at the DTC provided individual identifiers and attendance dates for DTC attendees.

All background variables used for propensity matching were taken from the PDHA. However, given the allowable time frame for completion, DTC attendees may have completed the PDHA form either before or after DTC attendance. For this reason, outcomes for assessing treatment effects are not taken from the PDHA. The study outcomes were taken from the PDHRA survey, which is typically completed three to six months after redeployment.

Data from the PDHA and PDHRA were requested for airmen deployed between January 2008 and August 2012, inclusive.[1] The Armed Forces Health Surveillance Center (AFHSC) merged DTC attendance information with PDHA and PDHRA records for a given deployment. They then removed all personal identifiers from the merged data file. AFHSC used a secure file transfer protocol to send the de-identified data to RAND for analyses.

The process of merging these data sources to create the analytic dataset resulted in a substantial loss of cases. This process is outlined in Figure 4.1. In particular, several DTC records were missing Social Security numbers (or contained only partial numbers), and about half had incomplete data on the dates of attendance (missing the date, year, or both). In many of these cases, however, we were able to infer an approximate date of DTC attendance because a class number had been recorded for some of the attendees, and most class numbers were assigned sequentially. In addition, there was no regular way to determine which participants were Air Force (and thus could be matched by AFSC to PDHA) and which were Marines. As a result of these issues, a substantial fraction of the total DTC attendees could not be linked to a PDHA by the AFHSC. In most cases, we do not know if these failures occurred because (a) the DTC attendee did not complete a PDHA, (b) the Social Security number recorded by the DTC was incorrect or incomplete, (c) the dates of DTC attendance (or imputed dates of attendance) were

Figure 4.1
Sample Accounting for DTC Attendees and Controls

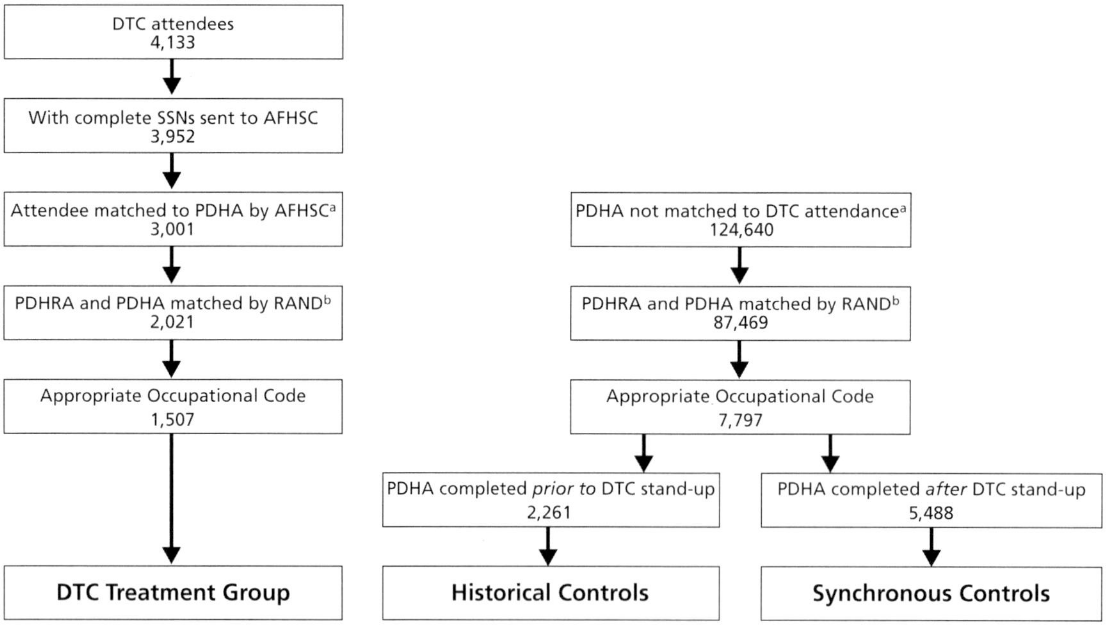

NOTE: SSN = Social Security number.

[a] A match based on having the same SSN and being the first PDHA completed after a date 30 days prior to the DTC attendance date. Total number of airmen PDHAs between January 2008 and August 2012 = 127,641.

[b] A match between a PDHA and PDHRA based on having the same unique ID, having deployment departure and completion dates within 30 days of one another, and not being a duplicate of another pair from the same deployment. Total number of airmen PDHRAs between January 2008 and August 2012 = 269,438.

RAND *RR918-4.1*

---

[1] PDHA and PDHRA data from Marines who attended the DTC were not available to the research team because our data use permissions were from the Air Force.

incorrect, resulting in a failure to identify a PDHA corresponding to the same deployment, or (d) the attendee was not an airman.

There were also minor losses for both the treatment and control groups caused by the need to match PDHA and PDHRA records from a given deployment. Airmen who did not complete both forms or did not accurately document the approximate dates of deployment could not be used in the analyses.

DTC Sample

The DTC sample comprised 1,507 enlisted airmen[2] who attended the DTC between the first quarter of 2010 and the third quarter of 2012 and who were in one of the following career fields: Tactical Air Control Party (1CF), Vehicle Operations (2T1), Vehicle Maintenance Control and Analysis (2T3), Explosive Ordnance Disposal (3E8), or Security Forces (3P0). Airmen in these career fields were generally scheduled to attend the DTC at the time they left for their deployments ("pre-identified" attendees), and these were the most common career fields among all DTC attendees. Thus, the sample largely excludes airmen who were command-referred to the DTC through a nominating process that is tied to their direct combat or trauma exposure. This exclusion was intentional, because it is plausible that some of the airmen who were command-referred were nominated specifically because their behavioral health problems had come to the attention of their commanders. Inclusion of such cases could have biased the results to make the DTC appear less helpful (or more harmful) than it actually is.

Control Sample

Selection of the control group was more complex. As discussed earlier, obtaining unbiased estimates of a treatment effect is dependent on successfully balancing the appropriate selection variables. To reproduce the treatment effects that would be achieved with an RTC, the control group should be composed of individuals who were eligible to attend the DTC, and they need to be matched to the actual attendees on any factors that might be associated with the outcomes.

For the DTC, we had two options for constructing the control sample: a historical control and a synchronous control group. Because the DTC did not exist before July 2010, the first option for a control group was to select individuals who returned from deployments prior to that date. If the DTC was not available, then the individual did not attend. We refer to this approach as the *historical control* approach. The second option was to use a control group of airmen for whom the DTC was available, but who for some reason did not (or could not) attend—we refer to this as the *synchronous control* approach. Both of these approaches have limitations, discussed below.

When using the historical control approach, the airmen in the control group are the target population the DTC was designed to serve but who could not attend because the DTC had not yet been stood up. While the selection mechanism is known, which is a desirable feature when conducting propensity analyses, this approach to estimating the treatment effect has a serious limitation. Because the control group deployed mostly in 2008 and 2009, but the

---

[2] Similar to Schneider, Bezdjian, and Burchett (2014), the analyses in this report were restricted to enlisted personnel. Officers have low rates of reported mental health problems and binge drinking within this data set, and they are more difficult to match using propensity scores due to their small numbers. In Figure 4.1, applying the listed career fields removed officers from both the treatment and control conditions.

treatment group deployed primarily in 2011 and 2012, the treatment effects are not separable from any broader changes in the Air Force or deployments over those years. That is to say, DTC treatment effects that are observed could be confounded with history effects.

The synchronous control approach does not confound treatment effects with history effects. Unfortunately, it has other limitations. It is made up of individuals who are not in the DTC analytic sample, even though many of them had been scheduled to attend the DTC. For example, Explosive Ordnance Disposal personnel (3E8) who deployed in 2011 and attended the DTC would be compared with other 3E8 personnel who deployed at the same time but did not attend. Because the DTC was scheduled to serve almost all 3E8 personnel returning from deployment over this period, we do not know the mechanism that caused those people to miss attending the DTC, nor do we know if such factors are captured in the available covariates. This approach could, for example, result in comparing airmen who attended the DTC to those from the same units who were medically evacuated from theater. Differences in PTSD across those groups may be caused by factors other than the DTC program. A related problem with this approach is that it limits the size of the control group to the small group of pre-identified DTC attendees who either could not attend or were deselected by their deployed commander and did not attend. This may reduce the statistical power to estimate the treatment effect, and it may make it difficult or impossible to closely match the DTC attendees with a synchronous control group (e.g., the control group has almost no 3E8 personnel). This problem is exacerbated by the problems with the DTC attendance records; approximately 25 percent of individuals who actually attended the DTC may have been included in the synchronous control group instead, because we could not identify them as DTC attendees due to missing/partial Social Security numbers or attendance dates.

While both approaches have limitations, the problems with using historical controls can be well addressed through additional analyses. Specifically, we can assess any history effects across the Air Force over the studied time period to determine whether those effects are possible confounds for the estimated DTC treatment effect. When history effects exist, we can explicitly test whether the DTC treatment effect is significantly different than those historical trends (an interaction effect, sometimes called a difference-in-difference test). As shown in Table 4.1, the DTC treatment effect is assessed by comparing DTC attendees with propensity-matched historical controls, while history effects can be estimated by comparing airmen who did not attend the DTC with their propensity-matched historical controls. Those two effects can be compared with each other to determine whether the estimated DTC treatment effects could be explained by broader trends in the Air Force over this time period.[3]

In summary, the historical control approach is our preferred approach to estimating treatment effects, because it offers the greatest power and the greatest comparability between the treatment and control groups. The problems with synchronous controls cannot be easily addressed by including a comparison to any historical trends. In the main body of the report, we present this historical control analyses. However, for comparison, we also completed a synchronous control analysis and present the results in Appendix A.

[3] This approach to eliminating confounding is often referred to as a difference-in-difference design.

Table 4.1
Study Design for Treatment Effects Estimated with Propensity Score–Weighted Historical Controls

Groups Being Compared	DTC Treatment Effect Estimation	History Effect Estimation
Treatment group (after DTC opened)	DTC attendees	Non-DTC Air Force Sample
Control group (before DTC opened)	Historical controls matched to DTC attendees	Historical controls matched to non-DTC Air Force sample

NOTE: DTC treatment effect is estimated by comparing outcomes between DTC attendees and their matched historical controls. History effects are estimated by comparing outcomes between recently deploying airmen who did not attend the DTC and their matched historical controls. The interaction effect tests whether changes in the outcomes over time for DTC groups are different than changes over time in the broader Air Force. The non-DTC Air Force sample is not matched to DTC attendees.

Key Measures

All background variables used for propensity matching were taken from the PDHA. These variables included demographic factors, career field, deployment characteristics (e.g., length), physical injuries, and deployment trauma. The PDHA is a mandatory survey that is completed within 30 days of redeployment. Given the allowable time frame for completion, DTC attendees may have completed the form either before or after DTC attendance. Because some airmen complete the form before they attend the DTC, outcomes for assessing treatment effects are not taken from the PDHA.

The study outcomes were taken instead from the PDHRA, which is typically completed three to six months after redeployment. We identified two PDHRA variables that, in our view, would be markers of poor reintegration: (a) the existence of social conflict, indicated by the respondent as "serious conflict with your spouse, family members, close friends, or at work that continue to cause you worry or concern" (dichotomous variable), and (b) frequency of binge drinking, defined as six or more drinks on a single occasion (range: 0–4, corresponding to never, less than monthly, monthly, weekly, daily). Although the PDHRA includes the AUDIT-C, the DTC program focuses on avoiding intoxication rather than drinking less frequently (indeed, DTC attendees are often taken to a beer garden as part of the program). Because the AUDIT-C is heavily affected by the frequency of drinking, this evaluation focuses instead on the binge drinking component of the AUDIT-C. This outcome better identifies drinking behaviors that put airmen at risk for health or legal problems and better aligns with DTC program goals.

We also included as program outcomes two PDHRA measures of psychological distress: (a) the number of different PTSD symptoms reported on the PC-PTSD (range: 0–4) (Prins et al., 2004), and (b) the total score from the PHQ-2 indicating frequency of depression symptoms (range: 0–6) (Kroenke, Spitzer and Williams, 2003). Although the DTC does not define itself primarily as a prevention program for diagnosable psychiatric disorders, it is designed specifically to reduce or prevent the behavioral health sequelae of deployment trauma, including distress related to the symptoms of depression and PTSD. It recruits only those airmen with highest exposure to deployment trauma and includes in its curriculum structured program elements that were originally designed for the purpose of reducing psychiatric symptoms or psychological distress (Adler et al., 2009). For this reason, we identified a reduction in post-deployment PTSD and depression symptoms as a goal of the program, in addition to reduced binge drinking and reduced social conflict.

It is worth noting that the PDHRA assessment used to measure key outcomes is not administered in a fully confidential manner. This web-based survey is designed to be used for both epidemiological research and as a screening tool to identify individuals who may benefit from health services. In particular, members who indicate a significant number of PTSD or depression symptoms are automatically referred to a mental health professional to perform an initial psychological assessment. This could lead to additional referrals and, ultimately, a formal diagnosis. It is likely that some symptomatic individuals underreport their true symptoms on the PDHRA to avoid talking with a mental health provider (although it is possible that others overreport symptoms because it could help them qualify for service connected disability benefits in the future). The magnitude of the response biases caused by this lack of confidentiality is not known but may be substantial. Because of the possibility of reporting biases, these measures should not be interpreted on an absolute level. However, they can be interpreted as measures of relative psychological distress when comparing across groups of airmen who took the assessment under similar circumstances.

Analysis

The analyses required several steps. First, we identified the enlisted DTC attendees who were from the targeted career fields. These airmen were likely to be attending the DTC because they were scheduled to attend, rather than because they were referred by their commander.[4] Second, we identified comparison individuals in those same career fields who completed a PDHA between January 2008 and July 2010 (the opening of the DTC). Third, we developed propensity weights that give increased analytic influence to those airmen in the control group who look most like the airmen who attended the DTC. This step results in a historical control group that has the same distribution of demographic, military, deployment history, and deployment trauma characteristics as those who attended the DTC (see Tables 4.2 and 4.3). Finally, we assessed the difference between the DTC and the weighted control groups for each outcome; we assessed these differences both with and without covariates.

The steps to investigate possible history effects were similar. The ideal group in which to investigate history effects would be composed of airmen who had some risk for PTSD or other deployment-related adjustment problems (like those who attended the DTC), but who were unlikely to attend the DTC. We first identified airmen who were in Air Force Specialty Codes (AFSCs) in which very few airmen attended the DTC. Among those, we included AFSCs in which there were at least ten deployments prior to the opening of DTC and ten after the opening. Finally, we eliminated those AFSCs whose members' average level of PTSD symptoms was lower than 0.08 (the median across career fields), to be more comparable to the types of airmen sent to the DTC. These exclusions produced a sample of 69 AFSCs. Those AFSCs accounted for 14,820 airman deployments between 2008 and 2012, with 5,177 of those deployments ending before the DTC stood up and 9,643 ending after. We calculated propensity weights using a similar method to that used in estimating the DTC treatment effect; we weighted the historical control group to have the same distribution of demographic, military, deployment

[4] Individuals who attended the DTC with unusual career fields (and thus were likely command-referred) did have worse outcomes on the PDHRA. Including those individuals as part of the treatment group results in less favorable estimated DTC treatment effects.

history, and deployment trauma characteristics as those whose deployment ended after the DTC opened. Thus, the comparison between these two groups is not affected by the DTC, since neither group includes DTC attendees, but it is affected by any broader historical trends in the prevalence of the key outcomes over the studied period.

To compute weights, we used the TWANG package in R (Ridgeway et al., 2014). This is a powerful and flexible program for deriving propensity weights. It uses an iterative, nonlinear, machine learning algorithm to obtain propensity scores. The control sample is then weighted by ($p/1 - p$), where p is the estimated propensity score (i.e., the predicted probability of being in the treatment group conditioned on the available information). This weighting method results in substantially better balance across groups than can be achieved with logistic regression or other common methods (Lee, Lessler, and Stuart, 2010; McCaffrey, Ridgeway, and Morral, 2004; Ridgeway and McCaffrey, 2007). The TWANG algorithm continues to add iterations that modify the weights (i.e., that increase the complexity of the model producing the propensity score) until the resulting weights show no further improvements in the balance across groups on the full set of background variables relative to the previous iteration. That is, it selects the final weights when the distribution of demographic, military, deployment history, and deployment trauma characteristics of the weighted control group is as similar as possible to the distribution in the treatment group. The propensity model included all variables contained in Tables 4.2 and 4.3, as well as all two-way and three-way interactions among those variables. The criterion used as a stopping rule was based on identifying the iteration that minimized the average Kolmogorov-Smirnov statistic comparing the distributions of treatment and weighted controls across all covariates.

We used Poisson regression to evaluate the difference in the outcomes between the treatment group and control group. Poisson regression is appropriate when the outcome of interest is measured on a count scale (e.g., symptom counts or frequencies). It is also appropriate for dichotomous variables when the prevalence is low, and the analyses are done with robust standard errors (e.g., Taylor Series Linearization). This statistical approach preserves the full information in the underlying scales, maximizing statistical power and precision, and it does not require that the outcome variables be arbitrarily dichotomized. The Poisson model tests effects estimated as the ratio of the means of the two groups (e.g., the average number of binge drinking episodes in the DTC group divided by the average number among the historical controls). This treatment effect can be estimated either with or without additional covariates. Covariates should be included whenever the propensity weights have failed to completely eliminate differences between the treatment and control groups (which can happen when the groups do not overlap sufficiently on the underlying distribution). Inclusion of these covariates results in "doubly robust" estimates that more closely mimic the treatment effects observed in an RCT. Covariates that are good predictors of the outcomes can also be included to increase precision in the estimation of treatment effects even when the weights achieved good balance across groups on those variables.

Finally, to determine whether the DTC treatment effects are confounded with history effects, we entered an interaction term in the Poisson regression. This statistically tests whether the ratio of means between DTC attendees and their historical controls on a given outcome is different than the ratio comparing the non-DTC Air Force sample and its historical controls.

That is, it is testing whether the DTC treatment effect is any different than trends on the same outcomes that occurred within the broader Air Force over the same period.[5]

We estimated Poisson models using the survey package in R 3.0.3 (Lumley, 2014). This package takes into account the effect of weights on both parameter estimates and their standard errors using Taylor Series Linearization.

Results

Balance Between Treatment and Controls

Tables 4.2 and 4.3 show the effect of propensity weights on the balance between the DTC attendees and their historical controls. Table 4.2 shows the demographic, military and deployment characteristics of the DTC group and the control group with and without propensity weights. Table 4.3 shows the deployment trauma experiences for the DTC group and the control group with and without propensity weights. The tables show either the mean (for ordinal variables) or percentage (for dichotomous variables) endorsing the category for each item. The *p*-value is the probability associated with the null hypothesis that the DTC and historical control groups have equal means on that measure. When the control group is well matched to the DTC group, the p-values will be larger, with very few values smaller than 0.05.

As shown in Table 4.2, historical controls were significantly older than DTC attendees. The propensity models reduced this discrepancy but did not eliminate it entirely. The gender balance of the DTC attendees was biased toward men compared with the control group; however, this difference was eliminated through the use of the propensity weights. DTC attendees had completed more deployments and spent longer on deployment than controls. The use of propensity weights substantially reduced these differences, but a small difference in total deployment length remained between DTC attendees and their weighted historical controls. Finally, there were considerable differences in AFSC. For example, 26 percent of DTC attendees were security forces (3P0), but over 60 percent of control group airmen were security forces. Propensity weights reduced this difference to a nonsignificant discrepancy.

The weights also improved balance on the PDHA variables measuring each airman's deployment trauma experiences and injuries (Table 4.3). Prior to weighting, 12 trauma variables showed difference between the DTC and control groups that were highly significant ($p < 0.01$), while none of the differences with the weighted controls were significant at the ($p < 0.10$) level. Achieving balance on these variables is crucial to the validity of the study because they are the best predictors of post-deployment behavioral health problems. Any differences between DTC attendees and historical controls on these deployment trauma variables would be an alternative explanation for differences observed in behavioral health outcomes. Prior to propensity weighting, DTC attendees were much more likely to report experiencing several types of deployment traumas and injuries relative to the historical comparison sample (Table 4.2). Of particular note is the variable assessing whether the respondent ever felt "in

---

[5] Thus, the current analyses deal with possible confounding variables using three analytic methods: propensity matching, covariate adjustment, and difference-in-difference design. Appendixes A and B contain additional methodological details about the analyses. In addition, they contain sensitivity tests that (a) compare a historical control versus synchronous control approach with estimating treatment effects and (b) investigate the sensitivity of findings to using alternative analytic methods.

Table 4.2
Demographic, Military, and Deployment Characteristics of DTC Attendees and Historical Controls Propensity-Matched to DTC Attendees

	DTC Attendees	Unweighted Historical Controls		Weighted Historical Controls	
	%/Mean	%/Mean	*p*-value	%/Mean	*p*-value
Age	28.2	28.8	<0.001	28.7	0.024
Gender (male)	93.3%	90.7%	0.003	92.9	0.257
Marital status			0.758		0.789
Married	55.0%	55.8%		56.0%	
Other	6.8%	7.2%		7.2%	
Single	38.1%	37.0%		36.8%	
Component			0.326		0.239
Active duty	92.6%	91.2%		93.4%	
National Guard	5.4%	6.2%		4.1%	
Reserves	2.0%	2.5%		2.6%	
Pay Grade			0.084		0.058
E-1–E-3	13.9%	11.0%		9.8%	
E-4	31.1%	31.0%		29.6%	
E-5	33.8%	33.7%		36.4%	
E-6	14.1%	16.1%		16.3%	
E-7	5.6%	6.8%		6.5%	
E-8–E-10	1.5%	1.3%		1.4%	
Total deployment length (months)	6.7	5.79	<0.001	6.54	0.040
AFSC			<0.001		0.239
1C4	10.7%	4.2%		10.9%	
2T1	30.9%	7.9%		27.7%	
2T3	5.2%	17.5%		7.0%	
3E8	26.9%	7.6%		26.0%	
3P0	26.3%	62.8%		28.4%	

NOTE: Unweighted historical controls are based on the subset of the Air Force population in one of the AFSCs listed. They are not representative of the overall Air Force. *N* = 1,507 DTC attendees; *N* = 2,261 historical controls matched to DTC attendees. *P*-value is for the null hypothesis that the mean/percentage among controls is the same as among DTC attendees.

Table 4.3
Deployment Trauma Experiences of DTC Attendees, Unweighted Historical Controls, and Historical Controls Propensity-Matched to DTC Attendees

	DTC Attendees	Unweighted Historical Controls		Weighted Historical Controls	
	%/Mean	%/Mean	*p*-value	%/Mean	*p*-value
Felt in danger of being killed?	38.8%	19.9%	<0.001	39.4%	0.811
Inspected destroyed vehicles?	25.9%	11.4%	<0.001	25.9%	0.995
Saw bodies or people killed or wounded?					
Yes, any	36.5%	20.2%	<0.001	34.9%	0.474
Enemy	18.9%	6.6%	<0.001	18.7%	0.920
Coalition	18.8%	9.7%	<0.001	21.7%	0.146
Civilian	15.1%	10.3%	<0.001	17.0%	0.266
Discharged weapon in combat?					
Yes, during this deployment	14.0%	3.4%	<0.001	12.4%	0.351
Land	11.7%	2.8%	<0.001	11.4%	0.840
Air	0.1%	0.0%	0.394	0.2%	0.894
Experienced event:					
Blast or explosion	29.9%	18.5%	<0.001	28.9%	0.621
Vehicular accident	6.3%	5.0%	0.092	7.2%	0.447
Fragment or bullet head wound	0.5%	0.1%	0.025	0.5%	0.844
Fall	9.8%	5.5%	<0.001	8.8%	0.435
Other Injury	7.9%	6.7%	0.164	8.2%	0.832
Immediately after experience above[a]:					
Loss of consciousness	3.6%	2.4%	0.226	3.6%	0.977
Felt dazed	14.7%	8.9%	0.002	12.1%	0.296
Memory loss	3.7%	2.1%	0.083	2.9%	0.517
Concussion	4.9%	2.6%	0.032	4.2%	0.673
Head injury	5.3%	3.8%	0.202	5.0%	0.857
Head injury causing problems[b]	65.5%	61.0%	0.312	66.7%	0.825
Injured during deployment	16.9%	13.2%	0.002	17.6%	0.684
Hospitalized during deployment	1.8%	2.1%	0.465	2.9%	0.111
Times seen by health care provider during deployment	1.16	1.12	0.652	1.24	0.497

NOTE: Unweighted historical controls are based on the subset of the Air Force population that matches the AFSCs of DTC attendees. They are not representative of the overall Air Force. *N* = 1,507 DTC attendees; *N* = 2,261 historical controls matched to DTC attendees. *P*-value is for the null hypothesis that the mean/percentage among historical controls is the same as among DTC attendees.

[a] Percentages reporting alterations of consciousness are given among those who reported an experience that may have caused a traumatic brain injury (TBI).

[b] Percentage is given among those airmen who indicate a possible TBI.

great danger of being killed" during the deployment. This item is the single best predictor of post-deployment PTSD and depression symptoms within the current dataset. DTC attendees were approximately twice as likely to have felt they were in danger of being killed during their deployment relative to the unweighted controls. After propensity weighting, however, DTC attendees were almost exactly matched to the historical controls on this variable and were not statistically different on all other trauma experiences during deployment.

Overall, the propensity weights dramatically improved the match between DTC attendees and their historical controls. The weighted comparison now more closely resembles an RTC in which there are few significant differences between the "treatment" and the "control" samples prior to treatment (approximately 1 in 20 variables will show a significant difference between treatment and control groups even with random assignment). However, some differences remained significant and may pose a threat to the validity of the study. To correct any biases caused by these imbalances, we included as covariates in the Poisson models variables that were still significantly different across groups even after weighting. We also included covariates in the Poisson model when a variable was a strong predictor of our outcomes. Including those covariates can improve the precision of our estimates even when groups are balanced on that factor. The following items were included as covariates: age, marital status, AFSC, pay grade, deployment length, number of deployments, and whether the respondent felt in danger of being killed during deployment.

Effect of the DTC on Post-Deployment Psychological Health

Table 4.4 shows the outcome means and 95 percent confidence intervals for the DTC attendees and the historical control group weighted to match to the DTC attendees. The differences between DTC attendees and their historical controls are small and not statistically significant for PTSD symptom counts, depression symptom frequency, and incidence of social conflict. For binge drinking, the mean for the DTC attendees is approximately 25 percent lower than the rate for their historical controls. While there is no evidence of a DTC treatment effect for PTSD or depression symptoms, there is a difference in binge drinking consistent with a treatment effect.

These observed differences need to be interpreted in the context of broader historical changes in PTSD, depression, and binge drinking that may have occurred over the same period among airmen who did not attend the DTC. To assess these historical trends, we examined these outcomes over time among airmen who were in AFSCs that were *not* sent to the DTC. These effects assess changes over time in these outcomes within the broader Air Force. As discussed earlier, the non-DTC sample is taken from airmen who redeployed after DTC was operational within career fields that did not attend the DTC. As with the estimation of the DTC treatment effects, they are being compared with matched individuals in those same career fields whose deployments ended prior to the standing up of the DTC. Because neither of these groups attended the DTC, any differences between them can only be attributed to historical changes in these outcomes over time. Those results are presented in Table 4.5.

We observed no significant trends in PTSD, depression, or social conflict in the non-DTC Air Force sample over this period. Interestingly, there was a significant reduction in post-deployment binge drinking observed over this time period, even for those airmen who did not attend the DTC. Within the greater Air Force sample (i.e., non-DTC), the average binge drinking score was 21 percent lower in the time period after the DTC opened. This may reflect the effects of a systemic effort within the Air Force to reduce binge drinking or

Table 4.4
Group Means and Estimates of DTC Treatment Effect

	PTSD	Depression	Binge Drinking	Social Conflict
Mean of DTC attendees	0.35 (0.32, 0.38)	0.39 (0.36, 0.42)	0.44 (0.41, 0.47)	7.0% (5.7%, 8.4%)
Mean of historic controls matched to DTC attendees	0.34 (0.27, 0.42)	0.40 (0.34, 0.48)	0.59 (0.54, 0.64)	6.5% (4.8%, 8.8%)
Bivariate ratio of means	1.04	0.98	0.75	1.08
95% confidence intervals	(0.81, 1.34)	(0.79, 1.20)	(0.66, 0.84)	(0.76, 1.56)
p-value	0.738	0.818	<0.001	0.663
Adjusted ratio of means[a]	1.04	0.97	0.74	1.07
95% confidence intervals	(0.81, 1.32)	(0.79, 1.20)	(0.67, 0.83)	(0.76, 1.51)
p-value	0.766	0.801	<0.001	0.695

NOTE: 95 percent confidence intervals are given in parentheses. Social conflict means are multiplied by 100 and expressed as a percentage. The *p*-values test the null hypothesis that the ratio of the DTC mean to the control mean equals 1.

[a] Ratio is adjusted for age, marital status, AFSC, pay grade, deployment length, number of deployments, and whether the respondent felt in danger of being killed during deployment.

Table 4.5
Group Means and Estimates of History Effects over Study Period

	PTSD	Depression	Binge Drinking	Social Conflict
Mean of non-DTC Air Force sample	0.15 (0.14, 0.17)	0.31 (0.29, 0.33)	0.29 (0.28, 0.30)	4.7% (4.3%, 5.2%)
Mean of historic controls matched to non-DTC Air Force sample	0.14 (0.12, 0.17)	0.30 (0.27, 0.33)	0.37 (0.35, 0.39)	4.6% (3.8%, 5.4%)
Bivariate ratio of means	1.07	1.04	0.80	1.04
95% confidence intervals	(0.91, 1.27)	(0.91, 1.17)	(0.74, 0.85)	0.85, 1.26)
p-value	0.405	0.586	<0.001	0.727
Adjusted ratio of means[a]	1.09	1.04	0.79	1.03
95% confidence intervals	(0.93, 1.28)	(0.92, 1.18)	(0.74, 0.85)	(0.85, 1.25)
p-value	0.289	0.507	<0.001	0.741

NOTE: 95% confidence intervals are given in parentheses. Social conflict means are multiplied by 100 and expressed as a percentage. The *p*-values test the null hypothesis that the ratio of the non-DTC Air Force mean to the control mean equals 1.

[a] Ratio is adjusted for age, marital status, AFSC, pay grade, deployment length, number of deployments, and whether the respondent felt in danger of being killed during deployment.

other population-level changes. The magnitude of the decline in binge drinking among DTC attendees relative to their historical controls was not significantly different from the decline in binge drinking in the overall Air Force during the same time period. The adjusted ratios of means are 0.74 and 0.79 for DTC effect and history effect, respectively. Those ratios are not significantly different ($p = 0.386$).

Study Limitations

The current evaluation was limited in several ways that may restrict the conclusions that should be drawn from it. First, although we have outcome data from a large fraction of DTC participants, problems with the quality of the attendance records from the DTC may have introduced biases into our estimates. A nonrandom group of individuals have been dropped from the DTC group (but are included in synchronous controls); to the extent that missing a Social Security number or other data is associated with the outcomes, their exclusion may bias the results. There are also important limitations tied to our measures. We analyzed outcomes that were directly or indirectly targeted by the DTC and that were measured on the PDHRA (PTSD symptoms, depression symptoms, binge drinking, and social/work conflict). Although we found no evidence of beneficial effects on these outcomes, that does not preclude beneficial effects on some other, unmeasured outcome of interest. Similarly, the failure to find beneficial effects three to six months post-deployment does not preclude short-term effects in the first days or weeks of reintegration. It is possible that beneficial effects existed one week after the DTC but had dissipated by the time airmen completed the PDHRA. Finally, to the extent that other types of outcomes are considered key metrics for the evaluation of the program, additional evaluation may be needed.

Discussion

We found no evidence of significant psychological or behavioral health benefits attributable to the DTC on the measures assessed with the PDHRA. When compared with a carefully balanced historical control group, the observed differences in the number of PTSD symptoms, the frequency of depression symptoms, and the existence of social conflict were very small, and nearly identical to differences observed in the broader Air Force over the same period. While there was an improvement over time in the frequency of post-deployment binge drinking, this trend was present both among DTC attendees and the broader Air Force and cannot be attributed to the DTC program.

Because this evaluation used a large sample and doubly robust methods to estimate the treatment effect of the DTC, these effects were estimated with high statistical precision. The findings rule out with 95 percent confidence long-term clinically meaningful improvement in mental health symptoms caused by the DTC (i.e., we can reject the hypothesis that the program results in a 25 percent improvement in symptom severity or likelihood of social conflict). In contrast, while the study did not find a statistically significant causal effect of DTC attendance on binge drinking (even at a relaxed criteria of $p < 0.10$), the confidence intervals on the estimated effect did not rule out the possibility of a clinically meaningful benefit.

As noted earlier, these conclusions are subject to several limitations. For example, it is possible that the program might have benefits on the primary outcomes if outcomes had been assessed in the days after DTC attendance, rather than three to six months after attendance.

It is also possible that the DTC program may produce benefits on outcomes that were not assessed.

Comparison with Previous DTC Evaluation

Our findings differ from the findings of Schneider, Bezdjian, and Burchett (2014), who analyzed similar data (i.e., they used almost identical data sources, time periods, and sample sizes). They concluded that DTC attendance was associated with mental health benefits assessed using PDHRA outcomes. Like the current analyses, their study also used a propensity matching method. We have performed significant follow-up analyses to identify why the RAND study did not replicate the earlier DTC evaluation. These analyses are presented in Appendixes A and B. Appendix A investigates whether the different conclusions are due to the use of a historical control design in the RAND report. However, a synchronous control analyses closely replicated the effect estimated in the historical control analysis and found no significant effects of the DTC. Appendix B investigates other differences in our covariates, samples, and propensity weights. These analyses identified two issues that explanation the divergent findings: First, the weighted control group in Schneider, Bezdjian, and Burchett (2014) looks different from both our weighted control group, as well as their own DTC group, on a range of covariates. Specifically, the propensity weights on their control group did not achieve good balance on key predictors of post-deployment mental health—i.e., their weighted control group reported significantly greater trauma exposure than did the DTC attendees. The better outcomes observed among DTC attendees are consistent with the fact that those individuals had fewer traumatic experiences during their deployments relative to the non-DTC control group with whom they were compared. This lack of balance was noted by the authors, but their statistical analyses did not address these confounds when estimating treatment effects.

In the process of trying to replicate their findings, we identified a statistical problem with their analyses. Their tests of statistical significance are based on incorrect standard errors. The SPSS procedures used for their analyses do not accept *survey weights*, but treat the propensity weight as the *frequency of a given observation*. As a result, the *p*-values they present are computed using an assumed sample size in the control group that is not related to the actual level of statistical precision in their effect estimates. For these reasons, we view the findings of the current report as superseding the conclusions of Schneider, Bezdjian, and Burchett (2014).

CHAPTER FIVE

Conclusions and Recommendations

The DTC provides airmen who are returning from stressful deployments a brief reprieve from both the conflict and the stresses of home. In a four-day "pause" between zones, the DTC gives airmen an opportunity to rest, take stock of their deployment experiences, and prepare for reintegration. The program serves a group of airmen who are at significant risk for developing mental health problems following deployment. Invitees are limited to those who may also benefit from the programming elements that focus on debriefing adverse events and education on adaptive coping and help seeking.

The program's commitment to serving all identified airmen immediately on departure from the conflict zone requires the program's physical infrastructure to be scoped for peak use. This includes hotel-like facilities on base, meeting space used for DTC activities, and facilities for the permanent staff. Staffing is more flexible; during periods when DTC resources are in high demand, additional staff are flown to Germany on TDY for extensive training and to facilitate group sessions. Although cost estimates were not available, the structure and scope of the program suggests a substantial financial commitment from the Air Force.

Scientific Literature Supports Some DTC Practices, but Others Are Contraindicated

Although the DTC does not define itself as a prevention program for psychiatric disorders, it recruits airmen who, on the basis of their deployment experiences, are at risk for posttraumatic behavioral health problems. It also includes in its curriculum structured program elements that were originally designed for the purpose of reducing psychological distress (Adler et al., 2009). As part of this evaluation, we reviewed the various components of the DTC program and linked them to similar activities that have been studied in the broader scientific literature. The program comprises elements similar to several other programs: an R&R component, an after-action interview to provide feedback for leadership, a psychoeducational component on successful transitions from a deployment to home that is very similar to the Army's Battlemind program, and a Telling Your Story component that shares some elements with Battlemind debriefing but is most similar to several posttraumatic debriefing programs studied in civilian populations (i.e., group-based emotional processing of traumatic events). The Army Battlemind program has been shown to produce small reductions in PTSD symptoms, depression symptoms, and sleep disturbance symptoms post-deployment among those with combat experiences. Thus, the literature supports the theory that those elements of the DTC program that borrow from Battlemind may be beneficial.

The broader effects of psychological debriefing programs (i.e., a primary prevention program involving groups of nondiagnosed individuals discussing and emotionally processing stressful incidents) have been well studied in a variety of populations. Unfortunately, this type of programming has repeatedly been found to be either ineffective or harmful to participants. The World Health Organization treatment guidelines for traumatized populations, as well as the *VA/DoD Clinical Practice Guideline for Management of Post-Traumatic Stress*, specifically recommend against these programs because of the lack of efficacy and potential for harm. While detailed, one-on-one discussions of traumatic events have been found to be helpful for individuals who have developed PTSD, similar procedures are risky when used as a group-based prevention strategy for those who have not yet developed PTSD. Encouraging people *whose natural coping mechanisms are functioning well* to process the trauma in a new way may disrupt their natural (and effective) recovery strategies. In addition, the vicarious exposure to other peoples' trauma and emotional reactions may serve to re-traumatize individuals who had been coping effectively with their own memories of trauma. In short, our review of the scientific literature suggests that some elements of the DTC program are consistent with programs shown to improve behavioral health and psychological distress, while other portions of the program are contraindicated in this population.

Attendees Appreciate the DTC Program

This evaluation of the DTC also reviewed data from DTC satisfaction surveys. These surveys (designed by DTC staff and administered to attendees near the end of the DTC program) showed that most attendees had positive opinions of the program. Eighty percent believed that attending the DTC was a worthwhile experience, and 74 percent believed that they were better prepared for reintegration after completing the program. Attendees were particularly enthusiastic about the quality of the accommodations, the opportunity to spend time in Germany, and the balance in the schedule between R&R and structured activities. They also appreciated the DTC's highly engaged personnel. Suggestions for improvement included policy changes to make attendance optional or to limit required attendance to those who saw combat and to improve on-site transportation and loosen program rules.

The DTC Did Not Improve Measured Post-Deployment Outcomes

Satisfaction among attendees is an important indicator of the quality of a program. Without positive support from program attendees, even an effective program will have difficulty remaining in service. However, it is important to also consider whether the program produces better psychological and behavioral health among attendees. We used propensity score analytic methods to estimate the treatment effects of the DTC. We compared outcomes among DTC attendees to a control group of airmen who were similar on all measured background variables (including demographic factors, military experience, career field, deployment history, and deployment trauma). We compared these groups on PTSD symptoms, frequency of depression symptoms, binge drinking, and social conflicts, as assessed on the PDHRA, three to six months after the DTC program. We found no evidence of significant psychological or behavioral health benefits attributable to the DTC among airmen who attended on these outcomes.

There was an improvement over time in the frequency of post-deployment binge drinking, but this same improvement was found among all members of the Air Force over the studied period, not just those who attended the DTC, and should not be attributed to the DTC program.

Recommendations

Our recommendations for the DTC depend, to a large degree, on what specific goals the Air Force hopes to achieve with the program. Program materials and staff indicate that there are a large number of possible benefits from participation. While the program design and elements are justified primarily in terms of benefits for psychological and social outcomes after reintegration, there may be other goals and benefits that can justify the program, which were not directly assessed in this evaluation. Our recommendations for the way forward depend on whether the outcomes we studied (particularly PTSD symptoms, depression symptoms, alcohol misuse, and social conflict) are sufficient metrics by which to evaluate the DTC. If the Air Force views improving those outcomes as the primary purpose of the DTC, then we would recommend that the resources directed to DTC be invested in alternative programs or treatments that have been demonstrated to improve those outcomes. Specifically, we would make the following recommendations:

Recommendation A1

Close or redesign the DTC and avoid recreating the DTC for future conflicts using the existing procedures and programming. The failure to show beneficial effects of the DTC on post-deployment PTSD symptoms, depression symptoms, alcohol misuse, or social conflict suggests that continuing to invest in the current DTC model may be a poor use of personnel time and Air Force resources.

Recommendation A2

Invest resources in programs or treatments that have been demonstrated to effectively treat post-deployment PTSD symptoms, depression symptoms, binge drinking, or social conflict (see *VA/DoD Clinical Practice Guideline for Management of Posttraumatic Stress*) or into new, promising programs that the Air Force evaluates for beneficial effects. These new programs may still make use of the DTC facilities and include some similar procedures but should have meaningfully different programming or eligibility.

On the other hand, if Air Force leaders decide that other benefits, not assessed in this evaluation, can justify the DTC, we recommend that the program be restructured around those alternative goals. For example, the program may be worthwhile because it provides airmen with well-deserved R&R following a difficult deployment. Alternatively, it may be useful for capturing after-action information that can feed into improved training and tasking. Other goals might include stress reduction during homecoming, positive opinions of the Air Force, and retention in the service. If achieving some of these goals is a primary purpose of the program, our recommendations are as follows:

Recommendation B1

Revisit, formally document, and evaluate DTC program goals.

Recommendation B1a

Develop a revised concept of operations that identifies how the program design, staffing, eligibility, and location are structured to achieve the goals that have been identified. For example, if airmen R&R is a key goal, the concept of operations should be restructured around that goal rather than behavioral health outcomes following deployment trauma. The program materials could answer questions such as: Should the program be staffed primarily with mental health professionals? Should all activities be mandatory? Should eligibility be limited to trauma-exposed airmen? Should participant selection be done in a way that maintains full utilization of the staff and facilities? Should timing be modified so that participation does not delay post-deployment leave? How do the available activities map onto participant interests or preferences? Should the program allow spouses or dependents to participate?

Alternatively, the program may be justified in terms of after-action information generated in discussions with career field facilitators. If this is seen as a primary goal, program materials should answer program design questions such as: Should participation be limited to the four career fields with significant trauma exposure? Should the group facilitator travel to the unit rather than having the unit travel to Germany for group discussions? Should the program be staffed primarily with mental health professionals? How should the information collected by the program be structured and disseminated to maximize its value?

The current program materials identify how the program was designed to improve a range of behavioral health outcomes following deployment trauma. To the extent that the DTC is justified in terms of other outcomes, the program materials should explain how the design, staffing, eligibility, and location have been structured, or restructured, to achieve those alternative goals.

Recommendation B1b

Because there is evidence that the DTC does not significantly reduce PTSD symptoms, depression symptoms, binge drinking, and social conflict, modify the program to reflect these findings. Remove curriculum elements that have unsuccessfully targeted these goals and, therefore, that may not be a good use of program or attendee time and resources.

If DTC decisionmakers wish to continue to target these outcomes, identify and implement alternative evidence-based prevention strategies. For example, if reducing post-deployment binge drinking remains an important DTC target, discontinue the alcohol education in the current curriculum, and introduce evidence-based alcohol misuse primary or secondary prevention strategies (Dimeff et al., 1999; Hustad et al., 2010; Jonas et al., 2012; Larimer and Cronce, 2002, 2007; Management of Substance Use Disorders Working Group, 2009; White et al., 2010).

Recommendation B1c

Develop an evaluation plan to empirically assess the effect of DTC attendance on important program objectives. In addition to an outcome evaluation, it may be important to conduct a cost assessment to determine whether the DTC is a cost-effective strategy to achieve program goals. For example, it may be more efficient to achieve recuperation goals by outsourcing provision of R&R days to a civilian resort facility.

Recommendation B2

Even if improving behavioral health is identified as a key program goal, remove the contra-indicated program element of group processing of psychological trauma and develop policy to prevent its reintroduction.

Conclusion

During our visit to the DTC, it was clear that the program staff were enthusiastic and committed to their mission. In satisfaction surveys, the quality of the staff and the skill with which they approached their mission was noted repeatedly by airmen, who appreciated the opportunity to attend. However, many well-intended and well-liked programs prove to be ineffective. In many ways, the history of mental health prevention efforts could be summarized in the same way. It has proved extraordinarily challenging to reach the right people, at the right time, with the right intervention to prevent the negative consequences of trauma exposure. In light of these challenges, it is not surprising that few prevention programs have been found to have benefits on post-deployment PTSD, depression, binge drinking, and social conflict. However, these evaluations are key for promoting ongoing program modification and program development that can improve outcomes for those airmen who serve their country on difficult or dangerous deployments. A continued commitment to this goal may still yield positive outcomes, even as the structure of the program changes.

APPENDIX A

Outcome Evaluation Using Propensity Score Matching with Synchronous Controls

Control Sample

The investigation of DTC treatment effects using synchronous controls is based on the same sample of DTC participants as was used in the primary analysis contained in Chapter Four. However, instead of comparing the DTC participants with similar airmen who deployed in the past, in this analysis DTC participants are being compared with similar airmen who deployed during the same time period but who were not identifiable as a DTC attendee in the administrative records (see Figure 4.1).

Unlike the *historical controls* approach presented in Chapter Four, the *synchronous control* approach does not confound the DTC treatment effects with history effects (and, therefore, does not require additional analyses to identify history effects among non-DTC career fields). However, the synchronous control approach has other limitations that may undermine causal inferences. This control group is made up of individuals who are not in the DTC analytic sample, even though most of them had been scheduled to attend the DTC. For example, Explosive Ordnance Disposal personnel (3E8) who deployed in 2011 and attended the DTC would be compared with other 3E8 personnel who deployed at the same time but were not listed in the DTC attendance records. Because the DTC was scheduled to serve almost all 3E8 personnel returning from deployment over this period, we do not know the mechanism that caused those particular airmen to miss attending the DTC, nor do we know whether such factors are captured in the available covariates. For example, it is possible that airmen who were injured or had behavioral health problems are concentrated in the synchronous control group because their deployments ended earlier than scheduled. In such a case, differences in PTSD across those groups may be caused by those factors rather than the influence of the DTC program.

The use of synchronous controls may also result in airmen who attended the DTC being placed in the control group due to incomplete recordkeeping of DTC attendance. More than 4 percent of attendees listed in DTC records had missing identifiers and, therefore, could not be included in the sample of DTC attendees. Their PDHAs and PDHRAs are incorrectly included in the control group. An additional 20 percent of attendees were not matched to a PDHA using the information available, which could occur if their recorded identifiers were incorrect or incomplete or if they failed to complete a PDHA. Thus, some of those individuals are also likely to be incorrectly included among the synchronous controls even though they should have been included as DTC attendees. In short, the synchronous control approach is more difficult to interpret, because we cannot identify the mechanism that caused the airmen in the control group to not attend DTC (injury? reassignment? command request?). That mechanism may be related to PTSD, depression, and alcohol misuse outcomes. In addition, there is likely some number of individuals who are incorrectly assigned to the synchronous control group but who actually attended the DTC due to the limits of the DTC recordkeeping.

Analysis

To construct the synchronous control group, we identified individuals in the career fields automatically assigned to attend the DTC who completed a PDHA after July 2010 (the opening of the DTC) but who were not identified as having attended the DTC. We developed propensity weights that give increased analytic influence to those airmen in the control group who look most like the airmen who attended the DTC. This step results in a synchronous control group that has the same distribution of demographic, military, deployment history, and deployment trauma characteristics as those who attended the DTC (see Tables A.1 and A.2). Finally, we assessed the difference between the DTC and the weighted control groups for each outcome, including covariates when they were necessary or appropriate.

As with the historical control group discussed in Chapter Four, we used the TWANG package in R (Ridgeway et al., 2014) to compute weights that balance the characteristics of the treatment and the control group. The propensity model included all variables contained in Tables A.1 and A.2, as well as all two-way and three-way interactions among those variables. The criterion used as a stopping rule was based on identifying the iteration that minimized the maximum Kolmogorov-Smirnov statistic comparing the distributions of treatment and weighted controls across all covariates.

We used Poisson regression to evaluate the difference in the outcomes between the treatment group and control group. The Poisson model tests effects estimated as the ratio of the means of the two groups (e.g., the average frequency of binge drinking episodes in the DTC group divided by the average frequency in the synchronous controls). Covariates are included whenever the propensity weights have failed to completely eliminate differences between the treatment and control groups (which can happen when the groups do not overlap sufficiently on the underlying distribution). Inclusion of these covariates results in "doubly robust" estimates that more closely mimic the treatment effects observed in an RCT. Covariates that are strong predictors of the outcomes are also included to increase precision in the estimation of treatment effects even when the weights achieved good balance across groups on those variables. We estimated Poisson models using the survey package in R 3.0.3 (Lumley, 2014). This package takes into account the effect of weights on both parameter estimates and their standard errors using Taylor Series Linearization.

Results

Balance Between Treatment and Controls

Tables A.1 and A.2 show the effect of propensity weights on the balance between the DTC attendees and their synchronous controls. Table A.1 shows the demographic, military, and deployment characteristics of the DTC group and the control group with and without propensity weights. Table A.2 shows the deployment trauma experiences for the DTC group and

Table A.1
Demographic, Military, and Deployment Characteristics of DTC Attendees and Synchronous Controls Propensity-Matched to DTC Attendees

	DTC Attendees	Unweighted Synchronous Controls		Weighted Synchronous Controls	
	%/Mean	%/Mean	*p*-value	%/Mean	*p*-value
Age	28.2	29.5	<0.001	28.9	0.018
Gender (male)	93.3%	89.3%	<0.001	93.9%	0.989
Marital status					
Married	55.0%	59.3%	<0.001	58.4%	0.378
Other	6.9%	8.9%		6.9%	
Single	38.2%	31.8%		34.7%	
Component					
Active duty	92.6%	91.3%	0.267	92.5%	0.999
National Guard	5.4%	6.5%		5.5%	
Reserves	2.0%	2.2%		2.0%	
Pay grade					
E-1–E-3	13.9%	3.8%	<0.001	11.3%	0.122
E-4	31.1%	29.5%		28.0%	
E-5	33.8%	40.3%		35.0%	
E-6	14.1%	16.9%		15.1%	
E-7	5.6%	8.0%		9.3%	
E-8–E-10	1.5%	1.5%		1.3%	
Total deployment length (months)	6.3	5.7	<0.001	6.2	0.386
Deployments in past 5 years	2.0	2.3	<0.001	2.1	0.009
AFSC					
1C4	10.7%	3.9%	<0.001	13.3%	0.006
2T1	30.9%	8.3%		28.4%	
2T3	5.2%	18.2%		7.0%	
3E8	26.9%	2.8%		19.9%	
3P0	26.3%	67%		31.4%	

NOTE: Unweighted synchronous controls are based on the subset of the Air Force population in one of the AFSCs listed. They are not representative of the overall Air Force. *N* = 1,507 DTC attendees; *N* = 5,488 synchronous controls matched to DTC attendees. *P*-value is for the null hypothesis that the mean/percentage among controls is the same as among DTC attendees.

Table A.2
Deployment Trauma Experiences of DTC Attendees and Synchronous Controls Propensity-Matched to DTC Attendees

	DTC Attendees	Unweighted Synchronous Controls		Weighted Synchronous Controls	
	%/Mean	%/Mean	*p*-value	%/Mean	*p*-value
Felt in danger of being killed?	38.8%	12.4%	<0.001	35.6%	0.239
Inspected destroyed vehicles?	25.9%	6.9%	<0.001	19.6%	0.011
Saw bodies or people killed or wounded?					
Yes, any	36.5%	13.7%	<0.001	33.5%	0.247
Enemy	18.9%	4.2%	<0.001	17.3%	0.483
Coalition	18.8%	5.9%	<0.001	16.7%	0.354
Civilian	15.1%	5.6%	<0.001	11.9%	0.062
Discharged weapon in combat?					
Yes, during this deployment	14.0%	1.8%	<0.001	11.9%	0.324
Land	11.7%	1.5%	<0.001	11.0%	0.727
Air	0.1%	0.0%	0.322	0.3%	0.489
Experienced event:					
Blast or explosion	29.9%	12.6%	<0.001	24.4%	0.028
Vehicular accident	6.3%	2.8%	<0.001	4.6%	0.077
Fragment or bullet head wound	0.5%	0.2%	0.075	0.5%	0.849
Fall	9.8%	4.4%	<0.001	8.7%	0.471
Other Injury	7.9%	8.1%	0.822	8.2%	0.811
Immediately after experience above[a]:					
Loss of consciousness	3.6%	2.2%	0.100	6.2%	0.411
Felt dazed	14.7%	9.5%	0.001	18.8%	0.299
Memory loss	3.7%	1.5%	0.009	3.7%	0.980
Concussion	4.9%	1.4%	<0.001	4.8%	0.981
Head Injury	5.3%	3.6%	0.097	6.5%	0.711
Head injury causing problems[b]	65.5%	59.3%	0.094	67.5%	0.718
Injured during deployment	16.9%	13.5%	0.001	17.1%	0.913
Hospitalized during deployment	1.8%	1.6%	0.659	2.7%	0.219
Times seen by health care provider during deployment	1.16	1.05	0.072	1.20	0.337

NOTE: Unweighted synchronous controls are based on the subset of the Air Force population that matches the AFSCs of DTC attendees. They are not representative of the overall Air Force. *N* = 1,507 DTC attendees; *N* = 5,488 Synchronous controls matched to DTC attendees. *P*-value is for the null hypothesis that the mean/percentage among historical controls is the same as among DTC attendees.

[a] Percentages reporting alterations of consciousness are given among those who reported an experience that may have caused a TBI.

[b] Percentage is given among those airmen who indicate a possible TBI.

the control group with and without propensity weights. The tables show either the mean (for ordinal variables) or percentage (for dichotomous variables) endorsing the category for each item. The *p*-value is the probability associated with the null hypothesis that the DTC and synchronous control groups have equal means on that measure. When the control group is well matched to the DTC group, the *p*-values will be larger, with very few values smaller than 0.05.

As shown in Table A.1, synchronous controls were significantly older than DTC attendees and had experienced more prior deployments. The propensity models reduced these discrepancies but did not eliminate them entirely. The gender balance of the DTC attendees was biased toward men compared with the control group; however, this difference was eliminated through the use of the propensity weights. Finally, there were considerable differences in AFSC. For example, 26 percent of DTC attendees were security forces (3P0), but over 60 percent of control group airmen were security forces. Propensity weights reduced this difference to a nonsignificant discrepancy.

The weights also improved balance on the PDHA variables measuring each airman's deployment trauma experiences and injuries (Table A.2). Prior to weighting, 15 trauma variables showed differences between the DTC and control group that were statistically significant at the $p < 0.05$ level (with 12 of those at the $p < 0.001$ level). In the weighted controls, only two of the differences were significant at the $p < 0.05$ level, with none at the $p < 0.01$ level. Achieving balance on these variables is crucial to the validity of the study, because they are the best predictors of post-deployment behavioral health problems (i.e., the study outcomes). Any differences between DTC attendees and synchronous controls in deployment trauma experiences would be an alternative explanation for any observed DTC effects on behavioral health outcomes. Prior to propensity weighting, DTC attendees were much more likely to report experiencing several types of deployment traumas and injuries relative to the synchronous control group (Table A.2). Of particular note is the variable assessing whether the respondent ever felt "in great danger of being killed" during their deployment. This item is the single best predictor of post-deployment PTSD and depression symptoms within the current data set. DTC attendees were approximately three times as likely to have felt that they were in danger of being killed during their deployment relative to the unweighted controls. After propensity weighting, however, DTC attendees were almost exactly matched to the synchronous controls on this variable and were not statistically different on all other trauma experiences during deployment.

Overall, the propensity weights dramatically improved the match between DTC attendees and their synchronous controls. The weighted comparison now more closely resembles an RTC in which there are few significant differences between the "treatment" and the "control" samples prior to treatment (approximately 1 in 20 variables will show a significant difference between treatment and control groups even with random assignment). However, some differences remained significant and may pose a threat to the validity of the study. To correct any biases caused by these imbalances, we included as covariates in the Poisson models variables that were still significantly different across groups even after weighting at the $p < 0.10$ level. We also included covariates in the Poisson model when a variable was a strong predictor of our outcomes. Including those covariates can improve the precision of our estimates even when groups are balanced on that factor. The following items were included as covariates: age, AFSC, pay grade, number of deployments, whether the respondent felt in danger of being killed during deployment, whether the respondent experienced a blast or explosion, whether the respondent experienced a vehicle crash, whether the respondent encountered civilian bodies or saw civilians killed or injured, and whether the respondent inspected destroyed vehicles.

DTC Treatment Effect

Table A.3 shows the outcome means and 95 percent confidence intervals for the DTC attendees and the synchronous control group weighted to match to the DTC attendees. The differences between DTC attendees and these controls are small and not statistically significant for PTSD symptom counts, depression symptom frequency, binge drinking, and incidence of social conflict.

Table A.3
Group Means and Estimates of DTC Treatment Effect

	PTSD	Depression	Binge Drinking	Social Conflict
Mean of DTC attendees	0.35 (0.31, 0.40)	0.39 (0.36, 0.42)	0.44 (0.41, 0.47)	7.0% (5.7%, 8.4%)
Mean of synchronous controls matched to DTC attendees	0.28 (0.23, 0.33)	0.37 (0.30, 0.44)	0.42 (0.37, 0.47)	6.1% (4.3%, 7.9%)
Adjusted ratio of means[a]	1.17	1.01	1.02	1.16
95% confidence intervals	(0.92, 1.45)	(0.82, 1.25)	(0.88, 1.17)	(0.81, 1.67)
p-value	0.215	0.927	0.708	0.409

NOTE: 95% confidence intervals are given in parentheses. Social conflict means are multiplied by 100 and expressed as a percentage. The *p*-values test the null hypothesis that the ratio of the DTC mean to the control mean equals 1.

[a] Ratio is adjusted for age, AFSC, pay grade, number of deployments, whether the respondent felt in danger of being killed during deployment, whether the respondent experienced a blast or explosion, whether the respondent experienced a vehicle crash, whether the respondent encountered civilian bodies or saw civilians killed or injured, and whether the respondent inspected destroyed vehicles.

Conclusions

We found no evidence of significant psychological or behavioral health effects attributable to the DTC among airmen who attended. When compared with a carefully balanced synchronous control group, the observed differences in the number of PTSD symptoms, the frequency of depression symptoms, the frequency of binge drinking, and the existence of social conflict were very small. These findings comparing DTC attendees to similar airmen deployed at the same time closely replicate the findings using historical controls presented in Chapter Four of the report.

The confidence intervals on the adjusted treatment effects suggest that any true beneficial effect is significantly smaller than a clinically small effect. For example, we can rule out with 95 percent confidence that the true treatment effect results in an 8 percent or greater reduction in PTSD symptoms. (This is because the lower confidence limit on the treatment effect is 0.92, which would represent an 8 percent improvement in DTC relative to controls).

APPENDIX B

Investigating the Differences Between the RAND and the Psychology Research Service Analytic Group's Analyses

The results of the current study do not replicate the findings of Schneider, Bezdjian, and Burchett (2014) or a preliminary analysis conducted by the same research group (Wirick, Garb, and Dickey, 2011) on a portion of this data. The Schneider, Bezdjian, and Burchett (2014) report was produced by the Psychology Research Service Analytic Group (PRSAG), and so we refer to it throughout this appendix as the PRSAG report. Their investigations also used propensity score matching to compare the DTC attendees with similar airmen who deployed at the same time (i.e., synchronous controls) on outcomes measured on the PDHRA. Unlike the current study, however, they found significant differences between the DTC attendees and the controls on depressive symptoms, posttraumatic stress symptoms, and social conflict. They concluded that DTC attendance appears to be protective of subsequent behavioral health problems. The goal of this appendix is to identify the differences in the data sets and in the analyses that might explain the substantially different findings across studies.

Differences in Data Sets

In general, the data sources are very similar but have a few notable differences. For both research groups, the list of DTC attendees and dates of attendance was provided by the DTC staff; the list of variables on which the treatment and control groups were matched was taken primarily from the PDHA assessment, which occurs ±30 days from redeployment; and the various outcomes were assessed on the PDHRA assessment, which occurs 90–180 days after redeployment.

Time Frame Studied

One difference in the data sets is that the PRSAG report authors used only data through calendar year 2011 in their study (18 months of DTC operation), although the DTC provided information about DTC attendees through April 2013. A rationale for this restriction was not provided in the report, but we infer that the researchers did not have access to one of the administrative data set for deployments ending in 2012 and excluded those deployments due to this missing data. The RAND analyses contained in Chapter Four and Appendix A of this report are restricted to deployments ending before August 2012 (26 months of DTC operation). This was selected because the PDHA and PDHRA instruments were revised for deployments beyond that date, including minor changes to both the covariates and outcome variables.

Because the studied time period used in the PRSAG report is a subset of the period in the current study, this difference can be investigated as the source of our discrepant findings. However, when we re-ran the analyses restricting the data to deployments ending before January 1, 2012, the study findings did not change for either historical or synchronous control comparisons. Although the different time periods did not explain the discrepancy in findings across these studies, all further analyses in this appendix restricted the RAND data set to the time period used in the PRSAG report to better identify the source of the differences.

Source of Career Field and Country of Deployment Data

The only meaningful difference in data sources between the two studies are that the PRSAG report used administrative records to assess some variables. Most notably, the authors used the Defense Manpower Data Center (DMDC) Active Duty Personnel file and the Contingency Tracking System (CTS) to assess (a) the career field (AFSC) for each case in the PDHA and PDHRA data sets, and (b) the country of deployment. In contrast, we identified career fields and countries of deployment from variables in the PDHA, which asks respondents to indicate their "occupational specialty during this deployment" and to list the countries in which they operated during this deployment along with the months spent in each location. In our analyses, the "country of deployment" was a derived variable that reflected the country where the respondent indicated serving for the longest time during his or her deployment. The career field variable plays a very important role in defining the eligible sample. And both career field and country of deployment play an important role in matching the DTC attendees to the controls, because there were substantial differences between the DTC and control group distributions of career fields and country of deployment prior to propensity balancing.

In theory, differences in the source of these variables should have little effect on the results. In the PRSAG report, the authors balanced treatment and controls with respect to their versions of these variables; in our analyses, we balanced treatment and controls with our versions of these variables. Both should allow for valid comparisons, since the information contained in our different versions of these variables should be similar. In practice, however, this difference makes it very hard to precisely align our data sets to identify the source of discrepant findings. For example, our self-report version of AFSC from the PDHA has some missing data and requires some hand coding (e.g., respondents could write "3E8," "3E831," or "EOD," all of which refer to the same career field). This certainly results in some cases being removed from the eligible pool (for both treatment and controls) in our study who would have been included in the PRSAG report, which uses complete data AFSC from personnel files. On the other hand, personnel records of career field reflect training and qualifications, not necessarily the tasks performed during a deployment, and the PRSAG report allowed matches for either primary or secondary career fields. Thus, the career fields used in the PRSAG report will not always accurately represent the occupation or task performed by that individual on a given deployment. Thus, if an airman is tasked with driving trucks during their deployment but had an AFSC code other than vehicle operator (2T1), the self-report measure will more accurately capture his or her deployment experiences. Because having one of several specific AFSCs is an eligibility criteria for both studies, the fact that RAND does not have access to the same personnel records means that we cannot precisely align our samples; we have slightly different group sizes and slightly different eligible cases.

Within these constraints, we attempted to align the data sets to determine whether there were differences in the raw data across the two studies. Table B.1 contains the means and per-

Table B.1
Comparison of Covariates Across Studies for DTC and Control Airmen

	DTC		Control		Weighted Control	
	PRSAG	RAND	PRSAG	RAND	PRSAG	RAND
AFSC						
1C4	6.2%	8.8%	4.1%	4.8%	8.7%	11.0%
2T1	42.2%	34.6%	4.7%	7.5%	34.0%	30.5%
2T3	6.9%	5.8%	12.7%	19.7%	5.8%	5.7%
3E8	20.7%	28.3%	2.3%	3.1%	26.6%	31.0%
3P0	24.8%	22.6%	76.7%	64.9%	25.6%	21.8%
Country						
Afghanistan	20.0%	35.5%	20.6%	36.1%	18.8%	34.1%
Iraq	4.35%	41.0%	5.3%	34.9%	4.6%	45.5%
Kyrgyzstan	10.7%	0.5%	16.0%	5.5%	8.8%	0.4%
Kuwait	52.1%	22.8%	14.6%	12.3%	51.2%	19.7%
Qatar	13.0%	0.3%	43.4%	11.3%	16.6%	0.3%
Deployment trauma						
Experienced blast	24.6%	30.0%	14.2%	15.8%	33.5%	21.7%
Encountered dead/wounded	28.7%	34.7%	12.5%	17.1%	37.9%	38.5%
Discharged weapon	7.2%	12.8%	2.0%	2.2%	7.0%	15.1%
Felt in danger of being killed	35.0%	37.5%	12.2%	15.4%	41.1%	36.3%
Entered/inspected destroyed military vehicles	22.4%	26.5%	5.3%	7.4%	29.0%	27.8%

NOTE: PRSAG data taken from Table 21 of Schneider, Bezdjian, and Burchett, 2014.

centages of the key variables used to balance the treatment and unweighted control group in the PRSAG report (taken from Table 21 of that report), along with RAND estimates of those variables when that variable is in our data set.[1] Table B.2 contains the means and percentages for the primary outcomes, but does not present estimates for the unweighted controls because the PRSAG report does not provide unweighted estimates of the outcomes among the controls. For this table, we attempted to scale/score these variables in the manner described in the PRSAG report, which may differ slightly from what was used in Chapter Four and Appendix A, and have limited our data to the same time period.

[1] The only PRSAG covariates missing from the RAND data set were those derived from PDHA Question 16, which asked "Are you worried about your health because you were exposed to..." and then lists several different environmental factors. This variable was not requested by RAND because it is not clear whether it is measuring a deployment experience (which you would want to match treatment and controls) or a behavioral health outcome related to anxiety (on which you would not want to balance).

The two variables where the studies used different data sources show differences across the two data sets. Looking at DTC attendees, the differences in career fields are small, with the RAND data set having a slightly higher proportion of Explosive Ordinance Disposal (3E8) and a slightly lower proportion of Vehicle Operations (2T1). Each of these differences constitutes only about eight percentage points of the sample. For unweighted controls, the primary difference is a slightly lower proportion of the control sample who were Security Forces (3P0) within our study. In both studies, however, the DTC and unweighted control samples were unbalanced in the similar way on AFSC, with a much lower proportion of the control samples having specialty codes 2T1 and 3E8 and a much higher proportion of 3P0 relative to the DTC samples. This imbalance is slightly greater in the PRSAG data, but both are large effects.

In contrast to the modest differences across data sets in career fields, the differences in "Country of Deployment" variable are dramatic. In the RAND data, 75 percent of DTC participants reported spending the largest portion of time in either Iraq or Afghanistan during their deployment. In the PRSAG report, only 24 percent of DTC participants were coded as deployed to either Iraq or Afghanistan in the CTS data. Because the DTC was targeted exclusively at airmen who were exposed to significant risk of trauma, the country codes in the PRSAG report data are unexpected. A similar difference exists among controls, with 71 percent of the RAND control group reporting their largest portion of the deployment spent in Iraq or Afghanistan, but only 26 percent of the PRSAG control group indicating either of those countries.

Follow up conversations with RAND and DMDC programmers who work with the CTS file suggests that the "location country code" variable contained in the CTS file does not indicate the country of deployment, but rather is an indicator of how personnel traveled into or out of the U.S. Central Command region. That is to say, it reflects an airman's travel itinerary rather than the location of his or her deployment.

Other than those two variables that were taken from administrative records, the two data sets show relatively close agreement on the characteristics of DTC attendees. On the variables taken from the PDHA that were used to create matched treatment and control groups (shown in Table B.1), the RAND and the PRSAG studies have broadly similar characteristics. The RAND data set shows slightly more exposure to blast among DTC participants. That is generally consistent with the slightly higher proportion of the RAND sample that were from the EOD career field. The question "During this deployment, did you ever feel that you were in great danger of being killed?" is the best single predictor of mental health problems in our data and was very similar for the DTC group across the two data sets (35 percent versus 37 percent endorsement). The unweighted control groups in both studies showed much lower exposure to deployment trauma relative to the DTC groups, and these control group participants were extremely similar in the pattern of trauma exposure across the two studies.

Similarly, we can compare the key study outcomes for the PRSAG and RAND data sets (Table B.2) among DTC attendees. (We cannot compare the control groups, as Schneider, Bezdjian, and Burchett did not publish unweighted estimates of outcomes in the control group.) The distributions on these variables are nearly equivalent across the two studies. The RAND DTC sample has identical levels of depression symptoms and a fractionally higher percentage who endorsed PTSD symptom relative to the PRSAG DTC sample. These small differences are generally consistent with our data set's slightly higher proportion of attendees who were in career fields 3E8, the group that experienced the highest levels of those symptoms (see Schneider, Bezdjian, and Burchett, 2014, Table 15).

Table B.2
Comparison of Outcome Variables Across Studies for DTC Attendees and Weighted Controls

	DTC		Weighted Control	
	PRSAG	RAND	PRSAG	RAND
PC-PTSD items				
Nightmares	7.5%	8.0%	13.9%	9.4%
Avoidance	7.0%	7.8%	7.9%	5.0%
Hypervigilance	10.0%	10.3%	15.5%	10.9%
Detachment	7.1%	7.4%	11.9%	7.9%
PTS composite	14.5%	15.7%	19.8%	19.0%
PHQ-2 items				
Low interest or pleasure in activities	0.22 (0.53)	0.21 (0.51)	0.36 (0.60)	0.19 (0.50)
Feeling sad, depressed, or hopeless	0.15 (0.45)	0.16 (0.45)	0.32 (0.59)	0.19 (0.50)
Alcohol use				
Frequency of alcohol consumption	1.35 (0.89)	1.40 (0.89)	1.28 (0.84)	1.36 (0.90)
Frequency of binge drinking	0.41 (0.61)	0.43 (0.62)	0.41 (0.59)	0.41 (0.60)
Family conflict	9.5%	6.5%	17.4%	7.7%
Difficulty getting along with others due to emotional problems	1.20 (0.46)	1.20 (0.47)	1.25 (0.48)	1.22 (0.49)

In short, the two studies rely on extremely similar data sets. When we restrict the analyses to the same time frame and use similarly coded variables, we find very few differences across the data used in the two studies. The one substantial exception is that the PRSAG report "country of deployment" variable taken from the CTS is distributed very differently than the nominally similar variable that was self-reported by airmen and used in the RAND analyses. Perhaps more importantly, the treatment and control groups within the PRSAG study also have very different distributions on that "country of deployment" variable. Therefore, this particular variable played a very large role in the propensity analyses within the Schneider, Bezdjian, and Burchett study because their weights are attempting to balance the DTC group (a majority of whom were coded as Kuwait) with their synchronous controls (a plurality of whom are coded as Qatar). The only other differences across the data sets appear to be the consequence of RAND using self-reported career fields, which results in the loss of some cases who failed to fill in this open-ended question on the PDHA with a response that could be coded to one of the qualifying AFSCs. This resulted in the RAND data set having a marginally higher proportion of Explosive Ordinance Disposal (3E8) personnel in the sample relative to the PRSAG study, as well as marginally more of the types of traumatic events and mental health symptoms that are associated with that career field.

Differences in Analyses

There is nothing obvious about the characteristics of the data sets that explains divergent findings across these two studies. The characteristics of the DTC groups are very similar on key risk factors, and the differences between the characteristics of DTC attendees and the unweighted synchronous controls are also similar; in both studies, airmen in the unweighted control group experienced dramatically lower rates of deployment trauma than those in the DTC group.

Although the data used in the two studies was similar, the statistical analysis of those data differed in several ways. More specifically, both analyses compared the DTC group with a weighted control using propensity matching in which the controls were weighted by their model-predicted odds of being a member of the DTC group. However, the two analyses differed substantially in the model used to predict those odds. The PRSAG report used a standard logistic regression model with predictors that included AFSC, country of deployment, and eight types of deployment and trauma experiences (see Schneider, Bezdjian, and Burchett, 2014, Table 21). Our model used to predict those odds was based on a nonlinear, nonparametric prediction model (using the TWANG package in the R statistical program [Ridgeway et al., 2014]) and included many more covariates than were used in the PRSAG report analyses (adding gender, age, pay grade, length of deployment, number of deployments in the past five years, and a more detailed assessment of deployment experiences). Our model also includes all two-way and three-way interactions among those variables. Thus, our model attempts to create two groups that not only have the same proportion of EOD technicians and of airmen exposed to explosions, but the same proportion of EOD technicians who were exposed to explosions. These variables are shown in Tables 4.2 and 4.3 for the historical controls analysis and Tables A.1 and A.2 for the synchronous controls analysis. Thus, our analyses were designed to achieve equivalence between the treatment and control group across a much broader range of factors.

The use of the TWANG algorithm to produce the weights allows researchers to balance across more variables (including collinear variables) and generally produces better balance than logistic regression (Lee, Lessler and Stuart, 2010; McCaffrey, Ridgeway, and Morral, 2004; Ridgeway and McCaffrey, 2007). This is largely attributable to the fact that the TWANG algorithm uses an iterative procedure that directly optimizes the weighted covariate balance between groups. That is to say, the final model is the one that provides weights that give the most similar distribution across groups across all covariates, as judged by the Kolmogorov-Smirnov statistic. Logistic regression optimizes the discrepancy of the model-predicted values relative to the actual group membership, which may not yield the model parameters that would have maximized similarity between treatment and weighted controls. Having said that, the specific algorithm used to derive propensity weights is not, itself, important for the validity of the subsequent analyses. Any two propensity weighting methods are similarly valid, so long as both methods succeed in producing groups that, when weighted, are balanced on the same list of covariates.

However, ours and the PRSAG report's propensity weighting analyses did not achieve similar levels of balance. For both the historical (Chapter Four) and the synchronous control (Appendix A) analyses, our weights did a good job of creating equivalent groups. For example, of the 31 variables (40 degrees of freedom) on which we attempted to equate our DTC attendees and the historical controls, there remained three variables on which there was a difference between these groups at the $p < 0.10$ level of significance, and two at the $p < 0.05$ level of significance. This is almost exactly the level of balance one would expect in an experiment in which cases had been randomly assigned to treatment or control conditions. Balance for the synchronous control analysis (Appendix A) was also acceptable, although not as good as expected in a randomized control trial. Out of 40 tested degrees of freedom, five tests were significant at the $p < 0.05$ level, and two of those were significant at the $p < 0.01$ level. Additionally, our analyses used to estimate treatment effects were conducted in a manner that was robust to incomplete matching from the propensity weighting. Any matching variables on which there remained differences between the DTC and control group at the $p < 0.10$ level of significance after weighting were included as statistical covariates in the models used to estimate the treatment effect. This is referred to as doubly robust estimation and can reduce bias in estimates of causal effects due to imperfect propensity matching, as well as from some types of omitted variables (Funk et al., 2011; Lunceford and Davidian, 2004).

In contrast, the PRSAG report weights did not result in good balance between the DTC and control group, even on the limited set of variables on which the authors attempted to create equivalent groups. On more than half of those variables, the authors report significant differences between the DTC group and the propensity weighted control group at the $p < 0.01$ level. The direction of this mismatch is particularly problematic. After applying the propensity weights, the "matched" control group has higher levels of virtually all major risk factors for post-deployment mental health problems relative to the DTC group. Airmen in the weighted control group were significantly more likely to have experienced the following traumas during deployment: a blast/explosion, feeling in great danger of being killed, encountering dead bodies, and inspecting destroyed vehicles. The weighted control group also included significantly more EOD (3E8) personnel than the DTC group, the career field with the highest levels of trauma and post-deployment problems in the PRSAG report data. The better behavioral health outcomes that the authors observed among DTC attendees are consistent with the fact that DTC attendees had fewer traumatic experiences during their deployments relative to the "matched" control group to whom they were compared.

This particular pattern of difference is perplexing. Both data sets show the unweighted synchronous controls as having much *lower* rates of trauma exposure (and less likelihood of being a 3E8) than the DTC group. Instead of balancing the DTC and control groups on those variables, the weights in the PRSAG report overcorrect for these differences, yielding a control group with substantially *higher* rates of trauma exposure than the DTC group. Thus, the particular imbalance in the weighted data was entirely created by the weighting process. Taken from the balance table (Table 21) in the PRSAG report, the prevalence of having been "in great danger of being killed" in the DTC group is 2.9 times the rate found in the unweighted controls, but in the weighted controls it is 1.2 times the rate found in the DTC group. The prevalence of having been "exposed to human blood, body fluids, body parts, or dead bodies" in the DTC group is 3.4 times the prevalence in the unweighted controls, but the weighted controls have 1.7 times the rate found in the DTC. Averaged over the eight types of traumatic deployment experiences included in the PRSAG report propensity model, the prevalence rate of trauma exposure for the DTC group was 3.1 times the prevalence in the unweighted controls, but after weighting the prevalence in the control group was 1.3 times the exposure prevalence in the DTC. Said another way, the PRSAG report propensity weights gave airmen in the control group who had been "exposed to human blood, body fluids, body parts, or dead bodies" approximately 6.8 times as much weight as the non-exposed airmen; however, achieving perfect balance on that variable only required giving them 3.6 times as much weight.

This imbalance problem is compounded by the manner in which the PRSAG report modeled selection for the propensity model. To be included in the multivariate propensity model, the authors required each variable to have a bivariate effect size[2] above a criterion value when predicting both treatment participation *and* at least one outcome. However, bivariate screening is considered an extremely problematic method for building multivariate models (see Harrell, 2001, pp. 56–60), and propensity methods are highly sensitive to this type of model misspecification (Rubin, 1997). Specifically, Schneider, Bezdjian, and Burchett's model selection method excluded many variables that were associated with key outcomes (see Table 20), such as being injured during deployment. Brookhart et al. (2006), cited in the PRSAG report to support the authors' variable selection method, specifically advises against this approach, concluding, "variables that are unrelated to the exposure but related to the outcome should always be included in a PS [propensity score] model." (See also Lunceford and Davidian, 2004, pp. 2950–2951, for a formal statistical argument of why those variables should be included.) Because many risk factors associated with the outcomes were not included in the propensity model, it likely that the propensity weights created imbalance on those omitted variables. We know that the weights "overshot" the target values on many types of trauma even though the model was trying to avoid imbalance on those particular variables; it is likely that the overshoot was even larger for those variables on which the propensity model was not trying to maintain balance. Omitting variables that are associated with the outcomes can create situations where the treatment effect estimated without propensity weights is less biased than when estimated with propensity weights.

Although the failure to achieve good balance was acknowledged in the PRSAG report (pp. 70–71), there was no attempt to control for the remaining differences through additional statistical procedures (e.g., covariate adjustment). There was also no discussion of the fact that the particular imbalance between the groups is in the direction that creates a bias toward overestimating post-deployment problems in the control group and thus overestimating the benefits of the DTC. This bias occurs because the DTC attendees are being compared to airmen who have higher levels of most risk factors for post-deployment problems. That is, the bias caused by the balance failure of the propensity weighting is in the same direction as the substantive findings presented in the study.

In an attempt to better identify the precise features of the analysis that resulted in substantially different findings across studies, we tried to directly replicate the PRSAG report's analytic methods for deriving propensity weights. However, when we use the procedures outlined in the PRSAG report on the RAND data set, we get weights that achieve acceptable balance, although not as well-balanced as when using TWANG. The final column of Table B.1 contains the weighted characteristics of synchronous controls when we try to replicate the

[2] The PRSAG report used the phi-coefficient as an effect size measure throughout the report when examining the association between two dichotomous variables. The labels (negligible, small, medium, large) used in that report correspond to typical interpretations of Pearson or Spearman correlation coefficients; however, the phi coefficient is not distributed in the same manner as those statistics except when the two variables being associated happen to have identical means/proportions. Cohen (1988), who developed the nomenclature of small, medium, and large effects, did not use the phi coefficient as a measure of effect size for this situation, but suggested the use of the *h* or *w* statistics, while treatment outcome studies typically use prevalence, incidence, or odds ratios to express effect size in such cases. Phi coefficients < |0.10| can routinely correspond to "medium" or "large" effects under Cohen's criteria, as well as under common clinical criteria (e.g., an odds ratio of 5 between conditions). Some of the variables being excluded from the propensity model on the basis of having "negligible" effect sizes may be considered medium or large effects under more standard effect size measures.

PRSAG report analytic methods; the data were restricted to the same time period and propensity weights were derived from a logistic regression model with the same, reduced set of predictors.

These weights do not provide nearly as good balance as was provided by the weights in the synchronous control analyses presented in Appendix A; they balance on fewer variables and do not get the DTC and weighted controls as close to one another on the variables they do include. Using this method, the weighted control group had slightly fewer of some traumas than the DTC group (experiencing blast, being in danger of being killed) and slightly more on others (encountering dead and wounded, discharging weapon). Although it "overshot" the target on some of the traumas, it did not overcompensate in the manner seen in the PRSAG report balance table—i.e., the weights did not convert a control group with too little exposure to deployment trauma into one with too much exposure on all exposure variables.

Using this analysis method, the treatment effect estimates are somewhat closer to the effects reported in the PRSAG report. Comparing the RAND DTC and weighted control columns in Table B.2, one can see that the point estimate for the weighted control group is higher than the DTC group for the composite PTSD symptom measure and the family conflict measure. That is, they are now in the same direction as found in the PRSAG report (and the opposite of what we observed in both Chapter Four and Appendix A). However, neither of those effects is statistically significant,[3] and so we do not replicate the findings of PRSAG report even when we used its method for deriving weights.

We spent considerable effort attempting to track down why the propensity weights used in the PRSAG report yielded this particular pattern of imbalance, but we cannot definitively identify the cause. We have investigated several hypotheses and conducted additional analyses in R, SPSS, and Stata in an attempt to identify possible software differences. We have two reasonable hypotheses for these differences. One possibility is that there is an error in some of the programming used in the propensity analyses portion of the PRSAG study. For example, some cases may have been excluded during the propensity matching but were then included in subsequent analyses. This can easily happen when computing *average treatment effect for the treated* (ATT) weights due to missing data on predictors. This missingness selectively drops cases from the control group (because those individuals do not get a weight from the logistic regression model), but does not remove similar cases from the treatment group (because a weight is not required). This results in imbalance across the treatment and weighted groups.

Another possibility is that a difference in the underlying data caused problems for the propensity model used in the PRSAG report but the problem is not present in the RAND data. The one substantial difference in the data sets, the country of deployment variable, was highly associated with DTC attendance in the PRSAG study's data. Thus, it would play a large role in the logistic regression model used to estimate the propensity scores. The presence of this variable may have interfered with the ability of the propensity model to achieve balance. The PRSAG report propensity weights gave airmen in the control group with a Kuwait coun-

---

[3] The only statistically significant difference between the RAND DTC and weighted control columns in Table B.2 is for posttraumatic avoidance, with DTC showing more avoidance than controls. It is worth noting that the differences in this table should not be interpreted as good estimates of the treatment effect, since the treatment effects presented in Chapter Four and Appendix A achieve better balance on more factors and have more power to detect a true effect.

try code nine times as much weight, on average, as those who had a Qatar country code.[4] If airmen with a Kuwait country code also, on average, had higher levels of trauma than those with a Qatar country code, it may not be possible to balance on the country variable without producing a weighted control group with too much trauma exposure.[5] Unfortunately, further investigation into this hypothesis requires more information than was contained in the PRSAG report.

Differences in Significance Testing

In the process of trying to replicate PRSAG propensity weights and treatment effects, we identified a serious problem with the report's statistical analyses: The significance tests for all of the treatment effects presented in the PRSAG report are incorrect. This error occurs because the SPSS procedures used for the report's analyses do not accept *survey weights*, but instead treat the propensity weight as the number of individual cases who had a given observation (i.e., *frequency weights*). The limitations when using SPSS with survey weights are discussed in the SPSS user's manual.

Propensity weighting produces survey weights, rather than frequency weights. The standard errors for statistics estimated on survey weighted data are determined by (a) the number of observations in the group, (b) the variance of the normalized weights, and (c) the covariance between the weights and the variable in question. For example, two weighted data sets (N = 100) may each estimate that 10 percent of airmen have posttraumatic symptoms. But in one data set, the 10 percent occurs because 10 people, each given a weight = 1, had symptoms, while in the other data set the 10 percent estimate occurs because one person with weight = 10 has symptoms. Using survey weights will correctly indicate that the estimated percentage in the latter case, in which the estimate is highly dependent on a single observation, has much more sampling error than in the former. Our analyses take these factors into account and estimate the standard errors of the treatment effects using Taylor Series Linearization (implemented in the SURVEY package in R 3.0.3; Lumley, 2014.).

In contrast, frequency weights are interpreted as the number of cases who were independently observed with that particular pattern of data. Giving a case a frequency weight of 10 is identical to copying that case's data and pasting it nine times in the data set. The standard error of estimates using frequency weights is determined by the sum of the weights; specifically, the error is proportionate to the square root of 1/(sum of weights). Unfortunately, the sum of the weights for survey weighted data is arbitrary and has no relationship to the sampling error

---

[4] The propensity weights shifted the proportion with Kuwait and Qatar codes from 14.6 percent and 43.3 percent in the unweighted control sample to 51.2 percent and 16.6 percent weighted for Kuwait and Qatar, respectively (see Schneider, Bezdjian, and Burchett, 2014, Table 21).

[5] As discussed earlier, we believe that the CTS country code assesses some aspect of the travel itinerary for the deployment, rather than the primary deployment location. As such, the large proportion of DTC attendees with Kuwait codes relative to others in the same career fields may reflect the typical route used to transport airmen to Ramstein Air Base. That is to say, the high number of Kuwait codes among DTC attendees may be partially a consequence of the fact that they were scheduled to attend the DTC. Because almost all injured personnel evacuated from theater are also flown to Ramstein (on route to Landstuhl Regional Medical Center), DTC attendees may have travel itineraries that are similar to airmen who are medically evacuated from theater. Thus, the control group airmen with Kuwait country codes may have higher average levels of trauma than those with other country codes. If it is the case that the weighted control group has a high proportion of medically evacuated personnel, it would represent a fundamental confound in the design, since such individuals are generally not eligible for the DTC. We used a historical control design as the primary method to estimate treatment effect to minimize the possibility of confounds like these.

of statistics computed on the weighted data. Indeed, the sum of ATT propensity weights for the control group will always be equal to the number of cases in the treatment group (because the control group is being weighted by their predicted odds of being the treatment versus control group). Using frequency weights, the standard errors for statistics estimated in the control group (e.g., estimating the proportion who experienced any posttraumatic symptoms) are unrelated to data from the control group, but are determined based on characteristics of the treatment group.

In general, treating ATT propensity weights as frequency weights could result in standard errors that are either too high or too low, depending on the relative sample sizes across groups, the variance of the weights, and their association with the specific outcomes. We have attempted to investigate the direction of bias using the RAND data set by comparing standard errors computed correctly (as survey weights) to standard errors computed incorrectly (as frequency weights). In our data set, we find that standard errors are slightly larger on our outcomes when using the correct weights. Therefore, the *p*-values are too low when treating them as frequency weights. We cannot know for sure if the magnitude of bias is the same in the PRSAG report, since there are differences in the weights across studies. However, we believe that it is very likely that the *p*-values for the treatment effects given in the PRSAG report overstate the statistical significance of the effects.

Conclusions

Our analyses and those documented in the PRSAG report came to substantially different conclusions about the effect of the DTC on attendees. We found no effects of DTC attendance across a range of behavioral health outcomes, while the authors of the PRSAG report found that DTC attendees had better health than a weighted control group across several behavioral health outcomes. A detailed investigation of the two reports identified four substantial differences in data or methods:

- We replicated findings using both a historical control group (employing a difference-in-difference design to assess for confounding history effects) and a synchronous control group, while the PRSAG report used only a synchronous control design.
- While both studies included a "country of deployment" variable to create propensity matched treatment and control groups, the variables were substantially different. Our variable was based on self-report and indicated that a substantial majority of DTC participants were deployed to Iraq or Afghanistan. The PRSAG report version was based on administrative data and indicated Kuwait or Qatar as the country of deployment for the majority of DTC participants.
- The propensity weights used in the PRSAG study resulted in meaningful differences between DTC and weighted control groups across a range of deployment experiences associated with study outcomes. Specifically, the DTC group was compared with a "matched" control condition that had increases in deployment exposure to blasts/explosions, feeling in great danger of being killed, encountering dead bodies, and inspecting destroyed vehicles. Our propensity analysis achieved better balance across a wider set of covariates, and we estimated the treatment effects in a manner that is robust to imperfect balance.

- The PRSAG report incorrectly estimated the statistical significance of treatment effects due to the limitations of SPSS when using propensity weights.

Our assessment is that these latter two differences contributed directly to the divergent findings across studies. In short, the imbalance between treatment and controls found in the PRSAG report resulted in a statistical bias toward finding lower levels of post-deployment problems among DTC participants relative to controls. This problem is compounded by the use of statistical procedures that produced incorrect *p*-values, leading to an overestimate of the statistical significance of those treatment effects.

For these reasons, we view the current report as superseding the findings of the PRSAG report with respect to the effects of the DTC on post-deployment health and functioning.

Abbreviations

AFHSC	Armed Forces Health Surveillance Center
AFSC	Air Force Specialty Code
ATT	average treatment effect for the treated
CFF	career field facilitator
CTS	Contingency Tracking System
DoD	U.S. Department of Defense
DTC	Deployment Transition Center
EOD	explosive ordinance disposal
IED	improvised explosive device
MSM	mission set manager
OEF	Operation Enduring Freedom
OIF	Operation Iraqi Freedom
PC-PTSD	Primary Care PTSD Screen
PDHA	Post-Deployment Health Assessment
PDHRA	Post-Deployment Health Re-Assessment
PHQ-2	Patient Health Questionnaire
PRSAG	Psychology Research Service Analytic Group
PTSD	posttraumatic stress disorder
R&R	rest and relaxation
RCT	randomized controlled trial
TAC-P	tactical air control party
TBI	traumatic brain injury
TDY	temporary duty assignment
TF-CBT	trauma-focused cognitive behavioral therapy

TLD	third-location decompression
VA	U.S. Department of Veterans Affairs

References

Adler, A. B., P. D. Bliese, D. Mcgurk, C. W. Hoge, and C. A. Castro, "Battlemind Debriefing and Battlemind Training as Early Interventions with Soldiers Returning from Iraq: Randomization by Platoon," *Journal of Consulting and Clinical Psychology*, Vol. 77, No. 5, 2009, pp. 928–940.

Adler, A. B., B. T. Litz, C. A. Castro, M. Suvak, J. L. Thomas, L. Burrell, D. Mcgurk, K. M. Wright, and P. D. Bliese, "A Group Randomized Trial of Critical Incident Stress Debriefing Provided to US Peacekeepers," *Journal of Traumatic Stress*, Vol. 21, No. 3, 2008, pp. 253–263.

American Psychiatric Association, *The Diagnostic and Statistical Manual of Mental Disorders: DSM 5*, 2013.

Babor, T. F., and M. Grant, "From Clinical Research to Secondary Prevention: International Collaboration in the Development of the Alcohol Use Disorders Identification Test (audit)," *Alcohol Health & Research World*, Vol. 13, No. 3, 1989.

Benish, S. G., Z. E. Imel, and B. E. Wampold, "The Relative Efficacy of Bona Fide Psychotherapies for Treating Post-Traumatic Stress Disorder: A Meta-Analysis of Direct Comparisons," *Clinical Psychology Review*, Vol. 28, No. 5, 2008, pp. 746–748.

Bisson, J., and M. Andrew, "Psychological Treatment of Post-Traumatic Stress Disorder (PTSD) (Review)," *The Cochrane Library 1*, 2009.

Bisson, J. I., A. Ehlers, R. Matthews, S. Pilling, D. Richards, and S. Turner, "Psychological Treatments for Chronic Post-Traumatic Stress Disorder Systematic Review and Meta-Analysis," *British Journal of Psychiatry*, Vol. 190, No. 2, 2007, pp. 97–104.

Bisson, J. I., P. Jenkins, J. Alexander, and C. Bannister, "Randomised Controlled Trial of Psychological Debriefing for Victims of Acute Burn Trauma," *British Journal of Psychiatry*, Vol. 171, 1997, pp. 78–81.

Bradley, K. A., K. R. Bush, A. J. Epler, D. J. Dobie, T. M. Davis, J. L. Sporleder, C. Maynard, M. L. Burman, and D. R. Kivlahan, "Two Brief Alcohol-Screening Tests from the Alcohol Use Disorders Identification Test (Audit): Validation in a Female Veterans Affairs Patient Population," *Archives of Internal Medicine*, Vol. 163, No. 7, 2003, pp. 821–829.

Brewin, C. R., "Systematic Review of Screening Instruments for Adults at Risk of PTSD," *Journal of Traumatic Stress*, Vol. 18, No. 1, 2005, pp. 53–62.

Brewin, C. R., B. Andrews, and J. D. Valentine, "Meta-Analysis of Risk Factors for Posttraumatic Stress Disorder in Trauma-Exposed Adults," *Journal of Consulting and Clinical Psychology*, Vol. 68, 2000, pp. 748–766.

Brookhart, M. A., S. Schneeweiss, K. J. Rothman, R. J. Glynn, J. Avorn, and T. Stürmer, "Variable Selection for Propensity Score Models," *American Journal of Epidemiology*, Vol. 163, 2006, pp. 1149–1156.

Brymer, M., C. Layne, A. Jacobs, R. Pynoos, J. Ruzek, A. Steinberg, E. Vernberg, and P. Watson, "Psychological First Aid Field Operations Guide," National Child Traumatic Stress Network and National Center for PTSD, 2006.

Cohen, J., *Statistical Power for the Behavioral Sciences*, 2nd ed., New York: Lawrence Erlbaum Associates, 1988.

Deahl, M., M. Srinivasan, N. Jones, J. Thomas, C. Neblett, and A. Jolly, "Preventing Psychological Trauma in Soldiers: The Role of Operational Stress Training and Psychological Debriefing," *British Journal of Medical Psychology*, Vol. 73, No. 1, 2000, pp. 77–85.

Deahl, M. P., A. B. Gillham, J. Thomas, M. M. Searle, and M. Srinivasan, "Psychological Sequelae Following the Gulf War. Factors Associated with Subsequent Morbidity and the Effectiveness of Psychological Debriefing," *British Journal of Psychiatry*, Vol. 165, No. 1, 1994, pp. 60–65.

Defense Manpower Data Center, *Contingency Tracking System (CTS) Deployment File Baseline Report (as of December 31, 2012)*, 2013.

Dimeff, Linda A., John S. Baer, Daniel R. Kivlahan, and G. Alan Marlatt, eds., *Brief Alcohol Screening and Intervention for College Students (BASICS): A Harm Reduction Approach*, New York: Guilford Press, 1999.

Donabedian, A., "Evaluating the Quality of Medical Care," *Milbank Memorial Fund Quarterly*, Vol. 44, No. 3, Part 2, 1966, pp. 166–206.

———, "Methods for Deriving Criteria for Assessing the Quality of Medical Care," *Medical Care Review*, Vol. 37, No. 7, 1980, pp. 653–698.

Fertout, M., N. Jones, and N. Greenberg, "Third Location Decompression for Individual Augmentees After a Military Deployment," *Occupational Medicine*, Vol. 62, No. 3, 2012, pp. 188–195.

Funk, M. J., D. Westreich, C. Wiesen, T. Stürmer, M.A. Brookhart, and M. Davidian., "Doubly Robust Estimation of Causal Effects," *American Journal of Epidemiology*, Vol. 173, No. 7, 2011, pp. 761–767.

Garber, B. G., and M. A. Zamorski, "Evaluation of a Third-Location Decompression Program for Canadian Forces Members Returning from Afghanistan," *Military Medicine*, Vol. 177, No. 4, 2012, pp. 397–403.

Gonzalez, G. C., R. Singh, T. L. Schell, and R. M. Weinick, *An Evaluation of the Implementation and Perceived Utility of the Airman Resilience Training Program*, Santa Monica, Calif.: RAND Corporation, RR-655-OSD, 2014. As of April 4, 2016:
http://www.rand.org/pubs/research_reports/RR655.html

Hacker Hughes, J. G., N. Earnshaw, N. Greenberg, R. Eldridge, N. T. Fear, C. French, M. P. Deahl, and S. Wessely, "The Use of Psychological Decompression in Military Operational Environments," *Military Medicine*, Vol. 173, No. 6, 2008, pp. 534–538.

Harrell, Frank E., *Regression Modeling Strategies*, New York: Springer Science & Business Media, 2001.

Hobbs, M., R. Mayou, B. Harrison, and P. Worlock, "A Randomised Controlled Trial of Psychological Debriefing for Victims of Road Traffic Accidents," *British Medical Journal*, Vol. 313, 1996, pp. 1438–1439.1432.

Hobfoll, S. E., P. Watson, C. C. Bell, R. A. Bryant, M. J. Brymer, M. J. Friedman, and M. Friedman, "Five Essential Elements of Immediate and Mid-Term Mass Trauma Intervention: Empirical Evidence," *Psychiatry: Interpersonal and Biological Processes*, Vol. 70, No. 4, 2007, pp. 283–315.

Hoge, C. W., J. L. Auchterlonie, and C. S. Milliken, "Mental Health Problems, Use of Mental Health Services, and Attrition from Military Service After Returning from Deployment to Iraq or Afghanistan," *Journal of the American Medical Association*, Vol. 295, No. 9, March 1, 2006, pp. 1023–1032.

Horowitz, M. J., *Stress Response Syndromes: PTSD, Grief and Adjustment Disorders*, Northvale, N.J.: Jason Aronson, 1986.

Hustad, John T. P., Nancy P. Barnett, Brian Borsari, and Kristina M. Jackson, "Web-Based Alcohol Prevention for Incoming College Students: A Randomized Controlled Trial," *Addictive Behaviors*, Vol. 35, No. 3, March 2010, pp. 183–189.

Jonas, Daniel E., James C. Garbutt, Halle R. Amick, Janice M. Brown, Kimberly A. Brownley, Carol L. Council, Anthony J. Viera, Tania M. Wilkins, Cody J. Schwartz, Emily M. Richmond, John Yeatts, Tammeka Swinson Evans, Sally D. Wood, and Russell P. Harris, "Behavioral Counseling After Screening for Alcohol Misuse in Primary Care: A Systematic Review and Meta-Analysis for the U.S. Preventive Services Task Force," *Annals of Internal Medicine*, Vol. 157, No. 9, 2012, pp. 645–654.

Jones, N., H. Burdett, S. Wessely, and N. Greenberg, "The Subjective Utility of Early Psychosocial Interventions Following Combat Deployment," *Occupational Medicine*, Vol. 61, No. 2, 2011, pp. 102–107.

Kroenke, K., R. Spitzer, and J. Williams, "The Patient Health Questionnaire-2: Validity of a Two-Item Depression Screener," *Medical Care*, Vol. 41, No. 11, 2003, pp. 1284–1292.

Larimer, Mary E., and Jessica M. Cronce, "Identification, Prevention, and Treatment: A Review of Individual Focused Strategies to Reduce Problematic Alcohol Consumption by College Students," *Journal of Studies on Alcohol*, Suppl. 14, March 2002, pp. 148–163.

———, "Identification, Prevention, and Treatment Revisited: Individual Focused College Drinking Prevention Strategies 1999–2006," *Addictive Behaviors*, Vol. 32, No. 11, November 2007, pp. 2439–2468.

Lee, B. K., J. Lessler, and E. A. Stuart, "Improving Propensity Score Weighting Using Machine Learning," *Statistics in Medicine*, Vol. 29, No. 3, 2010, pp. 337–346.

Litz, B. T., M. J. Gray, R. A. Bryant, and A. B. Adler, "Early Intervention for Trauma: Current Status and Future Directions," *Clinical Psychology: Science and Practice*, Vol. 9, No. 2, 2002, pp. 112–134.

Lumley, Thomas, "Survey: Analysis of Complex Survey Samples," R Package Version 3.30-3, 2014.

Lunceford, J. K., and M. Davidian, "Stratification and Weighting via the Propensity Score in Estimation of Causal Treatment Effects: A Comparative Study," *Statistics in Medicine*, Vol. 23, No. 19, 2004, pp. 2937–2960.

Management of Substance Use Disorders Working Group, *VA/DoD Clinical Practice Guideline for Management of Substance Use Disorders (SUD)*, Washington, D.C., Department of Veterans Affairs and Department of Defense, 2009. As of May 10, 2016:
http://www.healthquality.va.gov/guidelines/MH/sud/sud_full_601f.pdf

McCaffrey, D. F., G. Ridgeway, and A. R. Morral, "Propensity Score Estimation with Boosted Regression for Evaluating Causal Effects in Observational Studies," *Psychological Methods*, Vol. 9, No. 4, 2004, pp. 403–425.

McNally, R. J., R. A. Bryant, and A. Ehlers, "Does Early Psychological Intervention Promote Recovery from Posttraumatic Stress?" *Psychological Science in the Public Interest*, Vol. 4, No. 2, 2003, pp. 45–79.

Milliken, C. S., J. L. Auchterlonie, and C. W. Hoge, "Longitudinal Assessment of Mental Health Problems Among Active and Reserve Component Soldiers Returning from the Iraq War," *Journal of the American Medical Association*, Vol. 298, No. 18, November 14, 2007, pp. 2141–2148.

Monson, C. M., J. L. Gradus, Y. Young-Xu, P. P. Schnurr, J. L. Price, and J. A. Schumm, "Change in Posttraumatic Stress Disorder Symptoms: Do Clinicians and Patients Agree?" *Psychological Assessment*, Vol. 20, No. 2, 2008, pp. 131–138.

Mulligan, K., N. T. Fear, N. Jones, S. Wessely, and N. Greenberg, "Psycho-Educational Interventions Designed to Prevent Deployment-Related Psychological Ill-Health in Armed Forces Personnel: A Review," *Psychological Medicine*, Vol. 41, No. 4, 2011a, p. 673.

Mulligan, K., S. Wessely, N. Greenberg, N. T. Fear, and H. Alvarez, "Post-Deployment BATTLEMIND Training for the UK Armed Forces: A Cluster-Randomised Controlled Trial," *Occupational and Environmental Medicine*, Vol. 68, Suppl. 1, 2011b, pp. A48–A49.

Nash, W. P., and P. J. Watson, "Review of VA/DoD Clinical Practice Guideline on Management of Acute Stress and Interventions to Prevent Posttraumatic Stress Disorder," *Journal of Rehabilitation Research and Development*, Vol. 49, No. 5, 2011, pp. 637–648.

National Center for PTSD, "Using the PTSD Checklist," 2012. As of April 4, 2016:
http://www.ptsd.va.gov/professional/pages/assessments/assessment-pdf/PCL-handout.pdf

Ozer, E. J., S. R. Best, T. L. Lipsey, and D. S. Weiss, "Predictors of Posttraumatic Stress Disorder and Symptoms in Adults: A Meta-Analysis," *Psychological Bulletin*, Vol. 129, 2003, pp. 52–73.

Pennebaker, J. W., and K. D. Harber, "A Social Stage Model for Collective Coping: The Loma Prieta Earthquake and the Persian Gulf War," *Journal of Social Issues*, Vol. 49, 1993, pp. 125–146.

Powers, M. B., J. M. Halpern, M. P. Ferenschak, S. J. Gillihan, and E. B. Foa, "A Meta-Analytic Review of Prolonged Exposure for Posttraumatic Stress Disorder," *Clinical Psychology Review*, Vol. 30, No. 6, 2010, pp. 635–641.

Prins, A., P. Ouimette, R. Kimerling, R. Camerond, D. Hugelshofer, J. Shaw-Hegwer, A. Thrailkill, F. Gusman, and J. Sheikh, "The Primary Care PTSD Screen (PC-PTSD): Development and Operating Characteristics," *Primary Care Psychiatry*, Vol. 9, 2004, pp. 9–14.

PRSAG report—*See* Schneider, K. G., S. Bezdjian, and D. Burchett, *Evaluation of the Deployment Transition Center*, Seaside, Calif.: Department of Defense Center–Monterey Bay, 2014.

Ridgeway, G., and D. F. McCaffrey, "Comment: Demystifying Double Robustness: A Comparison of Alternative Strategies for Estimating a Population Mean from Incomplete Data," *Statistical Science*, Vol. 22, No. 4, 2007, pp. 540–543.

Ridgeway, G., D. F. McCaffrey, A. Morral, L. Burgette, and B. A. Griffin, "Toolkit for Weighting and Analysis of Nonequivalent Groups: A Tutorial for the Twang Package," *TWANG Package Vignette*, 2014.As of April 22, 2016
http://cran.r-project.org/web/packages/twang/vignettes/twang.pdf

Roberts, N. P., N. J. Kitchiner, J. Kenardy, and J. Bisson, "Multiple Session Early Psychological interventions for the Prevention of Post-Traumatic Stress Disorder," *Cochrane Database of Systematic Reviews 3*, 2009.

———, "Early Psychological Interventions to Treat Acute Traumatic Stress Symptoms," *Cochrane Database Systematic Reviews 3*, 2010.

Rose, S., J. Bisson, R. Churchill, and S. Wessely, "Psychological Debriefing for Preventing Post Traumatic Stress Disorder (PTSD)," *Cochrane Database of Systematic Reviews*, No. 2, Art. No. CD000560, 2002.

Rothbaum, B. O., E. B. Foa, D. S. Riggs, T. Murdock, and W. Walsh, "A Prospective Examination of Post-Traumatic Stress Disorder in Rape Victims," *Journal of Traumatic Stress*, Vol. 5, 1992, pp. 455 -475.

Rubin, D. B., "Estimating Causal Effects from Large Data Sets Using Propensity Scores," *Annals of Internal Medicine*, Vol. 127, No. 8, Part 2, 1997, pp. 757–763.

Schell, T. L., and G. N. Marshall, "Survey of Individuals Previously Deployed for OEF/OIF," in Terri Tanielian and Lisa H. Jaycox, eds., *Invisible Wounds of War: Psychological and Cognitive Injuries, Their Consequences, and Services to Assist Recovery*, Santa Monica, Calif.: RAND Corporation, 2008, pp. 87–115. As of April 4, 2016:
http://www.rand.org/pubs/monographs/MG720.html

Schneider, K. G., S. Bezdjian, and D. Burchett, *Evaluation of the Deployment Transition Center*, Seaside, Calif.: Department of Defense Center–Monterey Bay, 2014.

U.S. Department of Veterans Affairs Office of Public Health and Environmental Hazards, *Analysis of VA Health Care Utilization Among Operation Enduring Freedom (OEF) and Operation Iraqi Freedom (OIF) Veterans*, in presentation citing the Contingency Tracking System deployment file baseline report, Defense Manpower Data Center, provided to the Environmental Epidemiology Service of the U.S. Department of Veterans Affairs Office of Public Health and Environmental Hazards by the Armed Force Health Surveillance Center December 6, 2010.

Uhernik, J. A., and M. A. Husson, "Psychological First Aid: An Evidence Informed Approach for Acute Disaster Behavioral Health Response," *Compelling Counseling Interventions*, VISTAS 200, No. 9, 2009, pp. 271–280.

U.S. Department of Veterans Affairs and U.S. Department of Defense, *VA/DoD Clinical Practice Guideline for Management of Post-Traumatic Stress*, 2010. As of April 18, 2016:
http://www.healthquality.va.gov/guidelines/MH/ptsd/cpg_PTSD-full-201011612.PDF

U.S. Air Forces in Europe, *Concept of Operations: Deployment Transition Center* [amendment to tmt haf1310014987], Ramstein Air Force Base: Germany, February 2014. As of April 22, 2016:
http://www.ramstein.af.mil/shared/media/document/AFD-141016-012.pdf

VA/DoD Clinical Practice Guideline for Management of Posttraumatic Stress—See U.S. Department of Veterans Affairs and U.S. Department of Defense.

Weathers, F. W., B. T. Litz, D. S. Herman, J. A. Husk, and T. M. Keane, "The PTSD Checklist (pcl): Reliability, Validity, and Diagnostic Utility," Annual Convention of the International Society for Traumatic Stress Studies. San Antonio: International Society for Traumatic Stress Studies, 1993.

Werber, Laura, Margaret C. Harrell, Danielle M. Varda, Kimberly Curry Hall, Megan K. Beckett, Stefanie A. Stern, *Deployment Experiences of Guard and Reserve Families: Implications for Support and Retention*, Santa Monica, Calif: RAND Corporation, MG-645-OSD, 2008. As of April 22, 2016:
http://www.rand.org/pubs/monographs/MG645.html

Werber, Laura, Agnes Gereben Schaefer, Karen C. Osilla, Elizabeth Wilke, Anny Wong, and Joshua Breslau, *Support for the 21st-Century Reserve Force: Insights on Facilitating Successful Reintegration for Citizen Warriors and Their Families*, Santa Monica, Calif.: RAND Corporation, RR-206-OSD, 2013. As of April 4, 2016: http://www.rand.org/pubs/research_reports/RR206.html

Werber, Laura, Jennie Wenger, Agnes Gereben Schaefer, Lindsay Daugherty, and Mollie Rudnick, *An Assessment of Fiscal Year 2013 Beyond Yellow Ribbon Programs*, Santa Monica, Calif.: RAND Corporation, RR-965-OSD, 2015. As of April 4, 2016:
http://www.rand.org/pubs/research_reports/RR965.html

White, Angela, David Kavanagh, Helen Stallman, Britt Klein, Frances Kay-Lambkin, Judy Proudfoot, Judy Drennan, Jason Connor, Amanda Baker, Emily Hines, and Ross Young, "Online Alcohol Interventions: A Systematic Review," *Journal of Medical Internet Research*, Vol. 12, No. 5, October–December 2010.

Wirick, Aaron, Howard Garb, and David Dickey, "Report on the Deployment Transition Center: Post-Deployment Outcomes," unpublished manuscript, 2012.

World Health Organization Mental Health Gap Action Programme, *Psychological Debriefing in People Exposed to a Recent Traumatic Event*, 2012. As of April 22, 2016:
http://www.who.int/mental_health/mhgap/evidence/resource/other_complaints_q5.pdf

Zamorski, M. A., and B. G. Garber, "Drivers of the Perceived Value of a Third-Location Decompression Program for Canadian Forces Personnel Returning from Afghanistan," *Military Behavioral Health*, Vol. 1, No. 1, 2013, pp. 4–12.

Zamorski, M. A., K. Guest, S. Bailey, and B. G. Garber, "Beyond Battlemind: Evaluation of a New Mental Health Training Program for Canadian Forces Personnel Participating in Third-Location Decompression," *Military Medicine*, Vol. 177, No. 11, 2012, pp. 1245–1253.